Overcoming Burnout
Naturally

D1530805

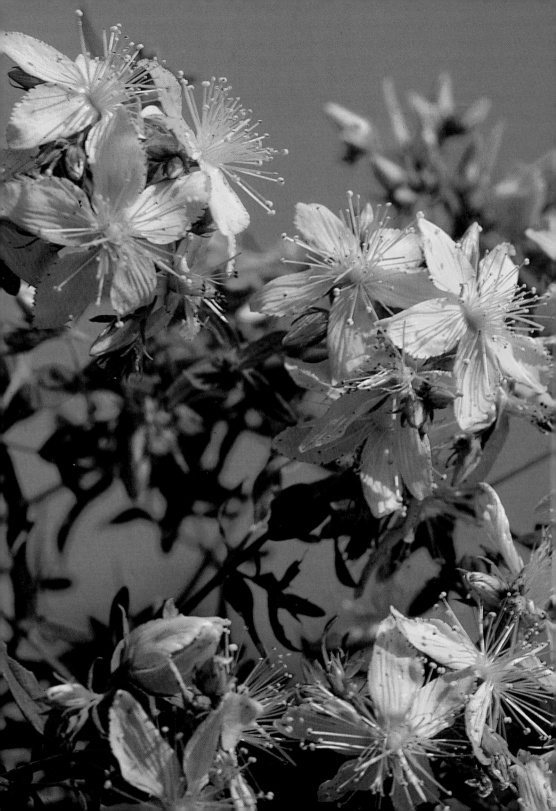

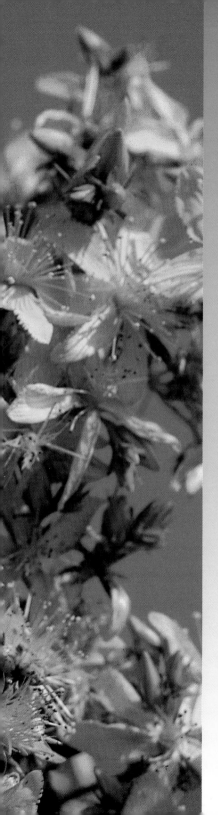

VINZENZ MANSMANN, M.D.

Overcoming Burnout
Naturally

Photo: Saint-John's-wort

Sterling Publishing Co., Inc.
New York

Picture Credits

Bavaria (TCL): front cover; Eisenbeiss, H.: page 7; Faltermaier, F.: page 81; Image Bank: pages 7, 10 (Alvarez, J.), 25 (Hamilton, D.); Jahreis, M.: page 80; Kimmig, U.: page 85; Kirchmaier, C.: page 77; Kracke, S.: page 42; Laux, H. E.: pages 2–3; Mauritius: pages 6 (Hubatka), 69 (SST), 84 (AGE); Okapia: page 17 (Kage, M.); Reinhard, H.: pages 2–3, 43; Schmitz, R.: pages 6, 72; Schneider, Ch.: pages 8, 54, 61; Tony Stone: pages 9 (Flies, C.), 11, 73 (Kaluzuy, Z.), 13 (Thomas, B.), 38 (Bosler, D.), 76 (Harvey, C.); Techniker Krankenkasse: page 35

Library of Congress Cataloging-in-Publication Data

Mansmann, Vinzenz.
    [Total ershopft mit naturheilmitteln zu neuer energie. English]
    Overcoming burnout naturally / Vinzenz Mansmann.
        p.   cm.
    "Originally published ... under the title "Total erschoptf mit naturheilmitteln zu neuer energie" - T.p. verso.
    Includes bibliographical references and index.
    ISBN 0-8069-2029-7
    1. Chronic fatigue syndrome Popular works. I. Title.
RB150.F37M3613 1999
616.0478–dc21
                                      99-36726
                                      CIP

10 9 8 7 6 5 4 3 2 1

Published by Sterling Publishing Company, Inc.
    387 Park Avenue South,
    New York, N.Y. 10016
Originally published in Germany under the title
    Total erschoptf mit naturheilmitteln zu neuer Energie
    and © 1997 by Gräfe und Unzer Verlag GmbH
English translation © 1999 by Sterling Publishing Company, Inc.
Distributed in Canada by Sterling Publishing
    C/o Canadian Manda Group,
    One Atlantic Avenue, Suite 105
    Toronto, Ontario, Canada M6K 3E7
Distributed in Great Britain and Europe by Cassell PLC
    Wellington House, 125 Strand,
    London WC2R 0BB, England
Distributed in Australia by Capricorn Link (Australia) Pty Ltd.
    P.O. Box 6651,
    Baulkham Hills, Business Centre,
    NSW 2153, Australia

Sterling ISBN 0-8069-2029-7

Preface

Chronic fatigue syndrome, also known as "burnout syndrome," afflicts millions of people around the world. It is estimated that as many as half a million people in the United States alone have a chronic fatigue syndrome–like condition. Women are clearly more prone to suffer from chronic fatigue than men. In fact, approximately twice as many women are believed to have the syndrome. The indications are there: constant exhaustion, the feeling of always being overtaxed, and difficulties concentrating—and not just at work. Is all this just a figment of the imagination—or are these the symptoms of an actual disease?

In this book, you will be introduced to the most common causes of the different types of fatigue, led through a diagnosis of your symptoms, advised regarding your choice of the right therapist, acquainted with the most important natural healing methods, and shown what you can do yourself in order to get back on your feet.

Vinzenz Mansmann, M.D.

CONTENTS

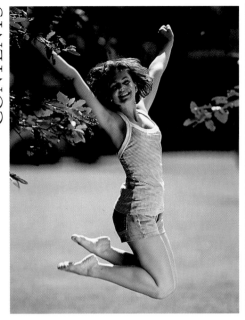

INFORMATION

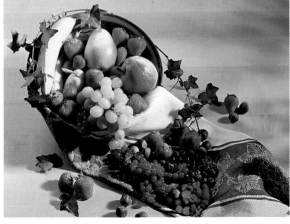

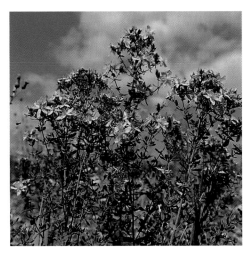
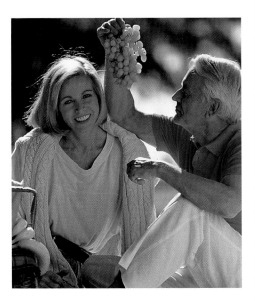

FATIGUE AS A DISEASE

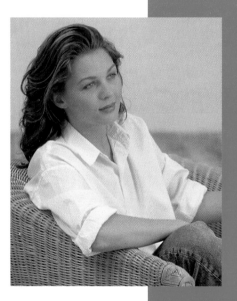

One thing is for sure: Under no circumstances should you excuse your fatigue as the result of overwork and too little time to recuperate. Why? Because if your most recent vacation had a lasting effect and you were fit and healthy, you would certainly not be reading this book. With this assumption in mind, let us start by taking a look at the various types of fatigue.

The Human Being: A Unity of Mind, Soul, and Body

Being happy is not merely the absence of pain but also has to do with feeling balanced emotionally. Even a young person with a healthy body doesn't necessarily feel this inner balance. For most of us, the daily bombardment of stimulation leads to an ever-increasing flood of restless thoughts. In addition, human beings are not content with just eating and sleeping but seek some deeper meaning in life in order to find happiness.

Mind	Our way of thinking, our thoughts
Soul	Our feelings and emotions
Body	Our carrier in this life on earth

The unity of mind, soul, and body

Exactly how does this complicated human being function? There is a mutual dependency among mind, soul, and body: One part cannot exist without the other parts. It is for this reason that troubling thoughts (such as those involving hate, anger, or rage) can lead to a lack of concentration, which can result in a sprained foot, for example. The subsequent pain can then affect the emotions: The physical pain causes unhappiness or misery, and thus the soul suffers along with the body. When all of a person's thoughts are focused on the aching foot, it is difficult to think of anything other than the physical pain.

As we approach every illness, in spite of being preoccupied with the pain we must ask ourselves the following questions:

❖ Why did the illness develop at this specific point in time?

❖ Which thoughts and feelings may have led to this illness?

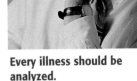

Every illness should be analyzed.

Listening to the Body

Deep inside, every person has a feel for the language of the soul, which tells us what is good for us and what is detrimental. When we ignore these silent signals, the suffering soul expresses itself through specific symptoms of physical ailments. In the case of a cold when your sinuses are blocked, try asking yourself what

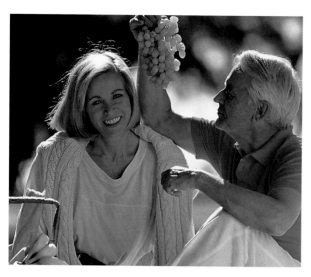

Correct nutrition helps to prevent burnout.

frustration could be the cause of the blockage. In the case of an ache in your limbs, the body knows that it cannot keep going on the way it has.

When you are exhausted after a meal, the digestive system is trying to tell you that it cannot digest so much food or such heavy dishes without withdrawing oxygen from other systems in the body. You have understood this message from the body correctly if you then ask yourself such questions as: Am I working too much, or am I under too much pressure? Am I getting enough sleep? Am I trying to achieve an unrealistic goal? How long will my body be able to bear this stress?

When you don't feel well, don't run immediately to a doctor or even to a practitioner of natural medicine. First, take some time to think about your interaction with your body. Take time to consider your feelings, your lifestyle, and what it is that your body is trying to communicate to you with its signals. If you are honest with yourself, you will have an even easier time than a doctor in discovering what changes you should make in order to stay healthy and lead a fulfilling life.

Various Types of Fatigue

Typical: Continuous psychological pressure, mourning, worries, trauma, depression, fear

In the case of your disease of fatigue, it is also essential to observe the signals with which your body is expressing itself. Therefore, at this point, I would like to introduce you to the various types of fatigue. When you compare these states with your own symptoms, please keep in mind that the divisions are arbitrary and it may well be that your symptoms fit into two or even three different categories. Later you will see that having a handle on your own type of fatigue can be of help in developing diagnostic and therapeutic strategies that will lead you through target-oriented processes in overcoming your fatigue.

Depressive Disorder Syndrome

There may be many different causes of a fatigue syndrome linked to depression. Psychology makes a distinction between reactive depression—which is a reaction to a certain event (such as a trauma)—and endogenous depression—which occurs (often unexplainably) without an obvious connection to any external cause. However, even when we are aware of the cause, it does not necessarily lessen the depression. Most of the time, the depression, regardless of its cause, brings on lasting pressure and uses up a great deal of energy:

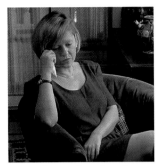

Some depressive disorders have an underlying organic cause.

❖ When a person close to us dies, we typically need a year of mourning in order to deal with the loss. Only after about a year and a half have passed would the mourning be regarded as pathological (that is, unhealthy).

❖ Divorce is also a loss. Overcoming this loss requires time too. The one who has been deserted is especially prone to depression.

❖ Most depressions are associated with fears. People who suffer from depression lack motivation and are often unable to carry out their daily tasks.

In order to overcome such a phase, the help of friends or a professional psychotherapist is usually needed. If you cannot detect an obvious cause for your depression, you should have your family doctor check to determine if you have an underlying physical disorder. Examples of such underlying causes of depression include a liver disorder, a metabolic disorder, or a hormonal imbalance. What follow are a few clues of which you should be aware.

Typical Symptoms of a Depression Caused by a Liver Disorder

❖ Lack of motivation in the morning
❖ Exhaustion following a warm lunch, to the point that you sometimes need to take a nap
❖ Feeling rundown
❖ Feeling exhausted
❖ Being extremely tired in the early evening (around 9 P.M.)
❖ Sleeping badly, not feeling refreshed in the morning when you wake up
❖ Waking up at 3 A.M. (the "liver time," according to the organ clock used in acupuncture, is 1–3 A.M., see page 47)
❖ Intolerance to different foods, suspicious of having various food allergies
❖ Digesting alcohol poorly, with its effects lasting for a few days
❖ Mood changes related to the season, with worsening effects in October/November and March/April

A Depression Caused by a Liver Disorder

People who suffer from a liver disorder are often misdiagnosed as having a metabolic disease, due to the fact that the liver does not have sensory nerves and we therefore cannot feel pain emanating from it. If you suffer from the symptoms that are highlighted in the box on page 11, you can conclude that your depression may well be related to a problem with your liver.

Depression during Menopause

Over the course of menopause, women often feel tired and depressed. However, I do not advise women to start treating these common manifestations of menopause with hormone pills or patches. After all, only 50 percent of the women who use these methods experience relief after the treatment. There are alternative solutions, which you can read about on pages 44–45.

Symptoms of a Menopausal Depression

❖ General weakness
❖ Profuse sweating
❖ Hot flashes
❖ Memory lapses
❖ Low motivation

A Potentially Suicidal Depression

When all impulses toward the external world are repressed and all feelings are reflected inward, depression runs the risk of turning into self-aggression. However, even professionals have a hard time diagnosing such cases.

The law in Germany allows a doctor to place a person under arrest for up to three days if that person expresses the intention of endangering his own life or the lives of others. This is a compulsory hospitalization, and it is done with the assistance of the police. Every year around Christmastime, such arrests escalate. Afterward, a judge is required to look into the matter.

Symptoms of a Potentially Suicidal Depression

❖ Compulsive fears
❖ Expressed intention of suicide
❖ Phobias, especially fears of heights, open spaces, or bridges
❖ Sudden dizziness in high places
❖ Depression after a long illness
❖ Depression after exhausting care for a relative
❖ Hopelessness, no thoughts for the future
❖ Despair

Overtaxed Nerves Syndrome

A person feels overtaxed and burnt out as the result of stress. This situation is familiar to most of us. But when we speak of stress, the matter is not as simple as it seems!

Good Stress—Bad Stress

Professor Selye, a pioneer in stress research, found in his experiments with rats that those that were raised in a completely stress-free environment were retarded in both their physical and emotional development, and showed evidence of being timid and distraught. Human beings also become stunted in their development if there are no stresses in their lives. Stress provides for a healthy level of flexibility. Stress in "normal doses" keeps us supple. Still, every person has a different limit of how much stress he or she can bear. We should know our own limits and not go beyond them too often. It also makes sense to distinguish between positive stress and negative stress. The increased heart rate before a date is an example of positive stress. Hatred, anger, rage, and jealousy are all examples of negative stress.

How Stress Becomes Overtaxing

Every stressful situation brings out physical reactions that worsen as the stress increases:

❖ **Initial reaction.** Stress makes us initially more mobile. The stress hormone adrenaline speeds up our circulation, and we become very alert and ready to take on any challenge.

❖ **The resistance stage.** The immune system becomes much stronger than it is under normal circumstances. There is a certain element of addiction to this kind of stress, which ends up strengthening our adaptability and our resistance.

❖ **The fatigue stage.** After long or intense periods of stress, the addiction element, mentioned above, is no longer felt, and eventually the stress leads to a state of burnout. During this stage, the immune system becomes drastically weaker than usual and illnesses cannot heal by themselves any longer. They settle in and become chronic. Such a situation can cause lasting damage.

Typical: Stress, too much work, too much stimulation, migraines, fears

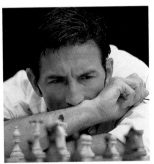

"Good" stress: An exciting game of chess

Whether you are in a state of constant stress or being buffeted by a series of stressful situations, not having a chance to unwind will lead first to psychological edginess and eventually to physical illness. Both are signals from the body telling you that it cannot go on this way any longer.

Immune Deficiency Syndrome

Typical: Recurring infections, problems with the intestines and the liver

The principles of positive stress and negative stress are valid not only for the body as a whole but also for every single organ.

Local Immune Deficiency

When a particular organ is under increased stress beyond that which the rest of the body is subjected to (for example, as the result of an injury), the body immediately engages in fighting the local damage. It sends out defense cells, causes certain biochemical reactions, and ensures that the overall temperature of the body increases. The organ under stress is becoming infected. The degree of infection depends on the balance between those hormones that accelerate the infection and those hormones that block it.

Specific hormone glands (especially the pituitary gland and the suprarenal gland) release hormones in response to stress. These hormones spread the infection in correlation to the level of the stress. Therefore, it is clear that infectious diseases can be caused not only by viruses, bacteria, and fungi but also by stress.

The Psychological Meaning of Infections

Psychological stress, which affects the mind and soul, can cause complications similar to those brought on by physical stress. When you are unable to face certain decisions and instead choose to repress the unresolved issues, you run the risk of placing an organ under relentless stress until the organ eventually becomes infected. Therefore, a physical infection can be seen as a reflection of an unresolved conflict within the mind or soul. The spiritual problem makes its way into the body in order to look for a resolution. It is not by chance that certain organs react to particular problems. Take these examples:

❖ When you are irked, or "galled," but don't vent these feelings, the gallbladder may get infected.

"What gall!"

❖ If instead of a face-off you choose to avoid a necessary confrontation, an infection may settle in the sinuses.

❖ Conflicts concerning your position at work, or at home with your spouse or partner, may lead to an infection of the abdominal organs (prostate or ovaries).

Intestinal Flora and the Immune System

One of the consequences of excess stress that is often observed is the occurrence of intestinal problems resulting from immune deficiency. How does this phenomenon take place? The surface of the intestinal wall in an adult covers approximately 358 square yards (300 square meters) and is full of billions of healthy bacteria. This intestinal flora is the primary factor in the human immune system. It provides us with about 70 percent of our defenses against diseases. If this organ is weakened, the door is thrown wide open to all sorts of bacteria, viruses, and fungi. What are the factors that deplete the intestinal flora and result in a corresponding weakening of the immune system?

❖ A leading factor is improper nutrition, especially ingesting an abundance of sweets. Not only can eating too many sweets bring on a fungus infestation, but in children this can also increase their susceptibility to infections. Both are particularly prevalent around Christmas and Easter, when sweets are generally consumed in greater amounts.

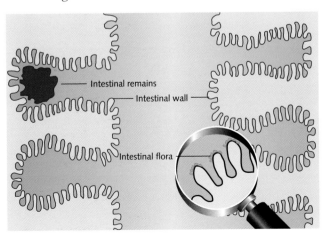

Intestinal remains

Intestinal wall

Intestinal flora

The surface of the intestinal wall is enlarged by the double indentation of the intestinal villus. This is where intestinal flora can be found. Intestinal flora is made up of billions of helpful bacteria. In addition, the remains of the digestive processes (that is, waste products) accumulate here.

❖ Antibiotics kill intestinal bacteria and thus weaken the body's resistance against incoming diseases. This is how putrid bacteria and fungi can find their way into the body.

Fungus Infections as a Sign of Immune Deficiency

Today, we live in a world where antibiotics are used so frequently that fungus infections have become a common problem (it is worth noting that penicillin has the active substance of fungus).

Fungus infections are caused by exaggerated disinfecting (the killing of good bacteria on the skin), antibiotics in the foods we eat (see page 25), and too many sweets in our diets, which create the perfect breeding ground for fungi. Once they have settled in, fungi are capable of doubling their numbers every twenty minutes. For example, a hundred cells can turn into ten million over the course of one night.

The most common type of fungus is the yeast fungus *Candida albicans,* which can settle into human skin and the mucous membrane. However, not every kind of fungus causes disease. Studies show that about 40 percent of the healthy human population is living with some harmless form of intestinal fungus and 75 percent of the human population with a weaker immune system is living with a fungal infection. But fungal infections are merely the tip of the iceberg. The underlying problem is a weakened immune system. Every year millions of people die from fungal infections and related complications.

How to Recognize a Fungus Invasion

❖ Thrush in the mouth, with white film on the gums (often occurring in infants), the tongue, or the teeth (appearing in people suffering from chronic diseases)
❖ White vaginal discharge (vaginitis)
❖ White film that is the result of a fungus infection between the teeth, between the fingers, or under the nails
❖ Itching eczema in the anal area

Typical Problems That Can Be Attributed to Fungi

❖ Flatulence, constipation, diarrhea
❖ Itching, redness, and sometimes a moist rash on the anus
❖ Stomachache, bad breath

❖ Exhaustion
❖ Lack of concentration
❖ Memory lapses
❖ Bad moods
❖ Cravings for sweets or foods rich in carbohydrates, such as bread and fruit
❖ Muscular shivers, followed by a feeling of intense hunger
❖ Seeing a shimmering in front of the eyes
❖ Being overweight, in spite of numerous diets
❖ Shortness of breath, stuffed nose as during colds, ear infections
❖ Muscular pain, stiff neck
❖ Pain in the joints, swollen joints
❖ Unclean-looking skin, reddened skin, pimples, dry skin, dull-looking and oily hair
❖ Musty body odor on hands and feet
❖ Fungus infections in the vagina, difficulties particularly before and after menstruation
❖ Urinary tract infections, prostate infections
❖ Diminished enjoyment of sex

If you suffer from several of these symptoms, not only should you make an appointment for a regular bowel examination (which often shows traces of intestinal fungi in healthy people) but also ask your doctor to take a special serological blood test.

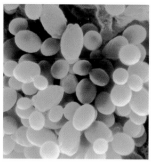

Only under a microscope can the form of the yeast infection *Candida albicans* be recognized.

Typical: Low blood pressure, sensitivity to the weather

Circulatory Disorder Syndrome

Many people suffer from low blood pressure. Without taking a cold shower or exercising in the morning, they can hardly start their day. Only after 10 A.M. are they fully awake. Doctors differentiate between: a functional circulation deficiency, in which specific parts of the body, such as the muscles, hands, feet, or brain, do not get enough oxygen, and an orthostatic malfunction of the regulatory system, in which the blood

Symptoms of Low Blood Pressure

❖ Difficulty starting your day in the morning
❖ Dizziness after standing up or bending down
❖ Dizziness after standing for a long time
❖ Tendency to suffer from headaches
❖ Sensitivity to the weather—for example, the feeling of being in a daze when a strong wind is blowing
❖ Difficulty concentrating in the early morning
❖ Difficulty learning in the first classes at school

stems its flow in the legs during long periods of standing, sometimes causing dizziness.

When Is the Issue Actually Low Blood Pressure?

The heart pumps blood into the arteries, creating a strong flow, which can be measured with a sphygmomanometer. The sphygmomanometer measures an upper level, which is also known as systolic blood pressure. Afterward, the heart releases the pressure and fills itself with blood as it recuperates. At this point, the lower level, or diastolic blood pressure, is measured, which shows us the ability of the heart to recuperate. We must remember that, after all, the heart cannot take any real break and has to work from the day we are born until the day we die.

These values are examples of low blood pressure.

Low Blood Pressure	under mmHg	to
Women	100	60
Men	110	60
Children (varies according to age)	90–100	50–60

Connections can be drawn between blood pressure and various states of the soul or the personality. A low blood pressure value on the high end can be linked to a lack of mental energy and to low self-esteem. One on the low end can be connected to a lack of strength, poor memory, and impatience.

Common Symptoms of a Sinus Infection

❖ Morning congestion, hoarseness
❖ Frequent stuffed nose, runny nose, pressure in the upper jaw or the forehead, especially during changes in the weather
❖ Chronic bronchitis, reaching acute levels in the morning
❖ Headaches, while in the sauna or during landing while aboard an airplane

Sinus Infections as a Frequent Cause

Over the course of my many years in professional practice, I have observed that a common cause of low blood pressure can be the unnoticed occurrence of chronic sinus infections either in the jaw or in the frontal sinuses. Unfortunately, such chronic infections cannot be detected through ultrasound or X rays taken by an ear, nose, and throat doctor, so they often remain undiscovered for a long time and thus are not treated in a timely manner.

Hormone Imbalance Syndrome

Hormones are proteins with regulation responsibilities. They are created in various places throughout our bodies. Some of them have a direct influence on our vitality.

Typical: Problems with the thyroid gland, sex hormones, and the suprarenal gland

Malfunctioning of the Thyroid Gland

With chronic fatigue, it's always necessary to check to see if it is the result of a thyroid insufficiency. Even in simple cases, such as a lack of iodine in the diet, it is not unusual for this gland to produce too little of the thyroxin hormone, which is an essential factor in maintaining our daily energy levels.

A case of thyroid insufficiency can be recognized by the swollen appearance of the thyroid in the front of the neck. This problem can lead to an iodine-deficiency goiter. This goiter is most common in places where little seafood is eaten, because seafood is a good source of iodine.

Depression during Menopause

In some cases, menopause may already begin at the age of thirty-eight to forty. Heredity can play an important role in these developments, but so can an undiscovered ovary infection (symptoms of which include discharge and problems related to the menstrual cycle). These factors can lead to a deficiency of female hormones, which makes menopause arrive ten years earlier than it normally does.

The ramifications of menopause, which include hot flashes, extensive sweating, insomnia, and weight gain or weight loss, can all lead to depression and a lack of passion—even during sex. Women can have the status of their hormones checked by having a blood test administered by their gynecologists. This hormone status report would tell them whether they have a menopausal hormone deficiency or not.

Advice

Pregnant women should have the level of their thyroid gland monitored regularly by their gynecologists. An iodine deficiency during pregnancy could impair the healthy development and subsequent growth of the brain of the embryo.

Out-of-the-Ordinary Hormonal Disorders

Due to the complex mechanisms of the various hormones in our bodies, disorders involving other hormones may lead to fatigue. In rare cases, the cause of the fatigue could be the malfunctioning of the parathyroid gland (hypoparathyroidism, usually as a result of a thyroid gland operation), the suprarenal gland (Addison's disease), or the pituitary gland (hypophysis, as often occurs in Cushing's syndrome). If your doctor expresses a suspicion that you might have any of the above problems, the exact nature of the medical condition needs to be verified.

Typical: Liver, gallbladder, pancreas, and intestinal problems

Metabolic Disorder Syndrome

All the organs that are related to the process of digestion have the role of turning our nutrition into energy. Health problems that are related to these organs result in a lack of energy (or fatigue).

Typical Symptoms of Liver Problems

❖ Extreme tiredness after a warm lunch, moderate tiredness after eating raw fruits and vegetables

❖ Digestive problems after eating a wide variety of foods, but especially fried foods

❖ Chronic constipation or the opposite—a tendency toward having diarrhea (especially after eating fatty foods)

❖ Poor sleep that is not refreshing

❖ Waking up between 1 and 3 A.M., which is the "liver time," according to acupuncture (see illustration on page 47)

❖ A tendency toward getting cramps in the calves, especially after drinking alcohol

❖ Very low tolerance of alcohol, suffering from headaches or exhaustion the following day

❖ Strong level of acidity in the body, with acidic sweat and frequent muscular cramps in the neck and back

❖ Worsening of the situation according to the time of year, especially in October/November and March/April

Liver Damage

We already know that pain in the liver is related to exhaustion; however, many patients with a liver disease are misdiagnosed or ignored, because it is not possible for us to actually feel pain in the liver and exhaustion is not clearly seen as a disease. In any case, a fat liver will be diagnosed, but a fat liver is the result of the liver's inability to deal with many years of an undiagnosed and therefore untreated liver disease.

In spite of the numerous intensive research studies carried out over the last few years, the biochemical processes of the liver, with its 370 components and more than 500 billion cells, are still only partially understood. It is therefore incorrect to believe that your liver is healthy if your doctor merely tested you for the three most common liver values (GGT, GOT, and GPT) and the results came back normal. Furthermore, these values often appear higher only when 80 percent of the liver cells are damaged.

If you have several of the symptoms that are highlighted in the box, you should suspect the possibility of a liver problem (see page 45).

Gallbladder Problems

The gallbladder is the keeper of the brownish-yellow gall fluids that are created in the liver. Unlike the liver, the gallbladder is surrounded by nerves and can spread acute colic pain. The entrance to the gallbladder can fall into spasms when a gallstone is being taken in or after we eat a fatty meal.

Gallstones do not appear by chance but are a result of many years of suffering with a malfunctioning liver. Therefore, the removal of the gallbladder does not guarantee the end of the acute colic pain, which issues from there, because the liver still continues to produce the wrong gall complex, which tends to give rise to crystals.

Gallstones: The result of many years of liver malfunction

If you have gallbladder problems, observe your bowel movements. If they are a light yellow color, then the gallbladder lacks brown gall fluids. If your bowel movements are whitish, this signifies the closure of the opening of the gallbladder.

Ailments of the Pancreas

A pancreatic disorder may lead to flatulence and tiredness after every meal. The pancreas not only produces insulin, which is lacking in diabetics (page 28), but also many other enzymes, which are responsible for the digestion of fat. A family doctor usually checks for two blood values (amylase and lipase), which change in the case of a disease.

Repeated instances of flatulence and tiredness after meals

Intestinal Disorders

New research shows that the intestines work at full speed especially in the late evening. Before we go to

The organs of the digestive system are important glands in human beings: In the case of fatigue, they can be the cause of the disease.

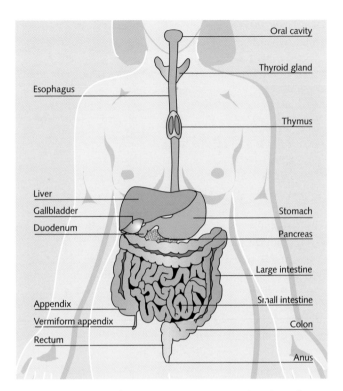

bed, the portion of the immune system related to the intestines (page 15) produces defense cells that destroy poisonous materials and transport foreign cells out of the body. Only when there are enough of these defense cells in the system does the brain release its natural sleeping aid, serotonin.

Therefore, disorders in the intestines are stronger during the night:

❖ In addition to the decreased ability to gain energy (due to the malfunctioning of the digestive system), the body's capacity to defend itself against diseases and poisons is reduced.

❖ Due to a lack of refreshing sleep, the body cannot fully recuperate from its efforts during the previous day and therefore keeps getting weaker and weaker.

Malnutrition Syndrome

Typical: Vitamin, mineral, trace element, and enzyme deficiencies

As unbelievable as this seems, in spite of a generally positive economic situation in much of the Western world, we are experiencing an increase in cases of malnutrition, which are typically accompanied by states of exhaustion.

Fast Foods and Excessive Fertilization of Agricultural Products

In spite of the abundance of vitamins in food, in the present age of fast foods the preparation of food is such that it often kills all the living vitamins that otherwise would be found. This can be the result of overcooking, microwave cooking, or keeping food warm for extended periods of time (as is the case with cafeteria food). Even simple decisions such as the choice to use white flour instead of whole-wheat flour can cause the body to ingest 90 percent fewer vitamins and minerals.

There are indications that our diets have deficiencies in such minerals as calcium, magnesium, iron, iodine, and zinc. One reason for these mineral deficiencies is worn-out and excessively fertilized soil. In fact, the amount of magnesium in wheat today is only 20 percent of what it was twenty-five years ago. In addition, the trace element selenium—the lack of which can lead to an immune system deficiency—has almost completely disappeared. Therefore, in many countries, the recommended levels for the most essential vitamins and minerals are not being reached.

The Five Stages of Vitamin Deficiency

❖ **First stage:** No symptoms yet; the body eats up its own reserves.

❖ **Second stage:** First signs of a reduced level of performance due to psychological stress or constant physical pressure.

❖ **Third stage:** Various symptoms, such as loss of appetite, weight loss, tiredness during the day, difficulty sleeping through the night, nervousness, edginess, susceptibility to infection, lower performance level.

❖ **Fourth stage:** Real deficiency syndromes, such as bleeding gums, resulting from vitamin-C and vitamin-K deficiencies, and problems seeing in the dark, resulting from a vitamin-A deficiency.

❖ **Fifth stage:** Complicated illnesses caused by a vitamin deficiency, like the ones that in earlier times would lead to death (such as scurvy, beriberi, and night blindness).

Free Radicals

The deficiency of the essential trace element selenium, mentioned above, has far-reaching implications. Selenium plays a major role in the fight against free radicals. The term "free radicals" refers to biochemical substances that, according to the latest research, are partially responsible for the spread of a number of afflictions today, including rheumatic fever, arteriosclerosis, high blood pressure, allergies, immune deficiency, diabetes type 1, Parkinson's disease, and even cancer.

Free radicals are created through many biochemical reactions in our cells, especially when there is not enough oxygen (as in cases of insufficient blood circulation). The body fights against free radicals with the aid of proteins that are rich in selenium (enzymes) as well as vitamins C and E and beta-carotene (which becomes vitamin A). For this reason, they are referred to as "free radical catchers," although the more scientific name is antioxidants.

Hypoglycemia (Low Level of Sugar in the Blood)

Hypoglycemia can be seen as another form of fatigue sometimes caused by malnutrition. People who are hypoglycemic have reactions to eating large amounts of food rich in carbohydrates (such as sweets). Within about an hour, the hormone insulin has used all the energy that was in the food, causing them to feel extremely enervated. With the drastic sinking of their blood sugar level, they not only feel exhausted but also shaky and fearful. Even though a piece of cake or some alcohol would temporarily remove these symptoms, this is not a permanent solution because obviously we can't eat sweets or drink alcohol every hour of the day.

In addition to malnutrition, a possible cause of hypoglycemia could be a disease of the pancreas or the liver or simply stress.

Typical: Being burdened by poisonous substances found in the home, medications, mercury from dental amalgams, and food allergies

Poison and Allergy Syndromes

The cells of the immune system combat internal poisons in the same way that they fight foreign attacks. For this reason, every battle against poisons or allergies weighs heavily on the immune system, weakens the liver, and robs us of a considerable amount of energy. The result is a deficiency in the immune system as well as fatigue.

Poisons at Home and in the Office

Chemical poisoning has become, for many of us, an unavoidable part of daily life. Chemical poisons are found in wood paneling, wood beams, carpets, walls, furniture, and window frames, as well as in leather covers on living-room furniture and in clothing. The poisons usually cause headaches, a reduced level of performance, tiredness after meals or any minor exertion, and chronic fatigue.

The danger that the poisons pose is that they sink into our systems over the years, even though they may not cause actual pain. Experience shows that people who have been so poisoned seek medical help at least five years after living or working in such an environment. It takes that long for the liver to no longer be able to detoxify the body and for the effects of this to worsen. Furthermore, it has been proven that these environmental chemical poisons damage the immune system.

Poisons in Food

Pesticides are known to be found in fruits and vegetables. Their purpose is to protect fruits and vegetables from insects, fungi, or bacteria. Not only do farmers use these pesticides, but amateur gardeners also spray their vegetables with them in order to get rid of

The Leading Poisonous Substances in the Home

❖ Lindane (an insecticide that is biodegraded very slowly and found in wood varnishes mostly used on wood beams, in leather, and even in clothing shipped long distances from Asia)
❖ Pentachlorophenol, or PCP (used as a wood preservative in wood varnishes and found mostly in treated wood)
❖ Formaldehyde (a preservative found in pressboard furniture and carpet glue)
❖ Various sorts of polychlorinated biphenyl, or PCB (a compound used in rubber joints and appliances for protection against fire and found mainly in public buildings, such as schools and concert halls)

The most tempting fruits have usually been sprayed with pesticides.

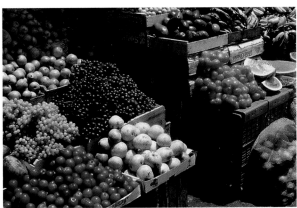

insects, snails, fungi, and weeds. In addition to pesticides, there are other hidden sources of poison. A good example of this is when oranges lie an entire week in lindane-treated wooden boxes aboard a ship.

We know virtually nothing about the influence of a wide variety of preservation methods on our health. For instance, when spices and other nutritional substances are treated with X rays, the effects are unknown. Have you ever had a tomato sitting in your warm kitchen for a month without rotting? Clearly it was treated with something.

Doctors believe that an allergy to penicillin, which sometimes occurs in people who never took penicillin in their lives, is the result of the large amount of antibiotics found in food, especially in pork. Due to lax slaughtering regulations, these medications are allowed to be administered to the animals up to three days before they are killed. At this point, although no trace of the antibiotics is found in the blood, we don't know if deposits are in the fatty tissue because this simply is not being checked.

Typical Symptoms of Problems Caused by Quicksilver

❖ Tiredness, sleepiness
❖ Mental edginess (a tendency to explode over minor issues)
❖ Depressive moods and a lack of passion
❖ Generally poor health, but without identifiable symptoms

Quicksilver from Amalgam Fillings

For dozens of years, amalgam fillings were considered harmless and inexpensive. But the quicksilver (also called mercury) can be released over the years in a variety of ways. The blood will spread it evenly throughout the body, and it will be deposited in the various organs, even the brain. According to my findings, quicksilver is released from the amalgam only when there is a high level of acidity in the body. This acidity can be caused by eating too much meat or too many sweets, by liver or gallbladder diseases, by gout (high levels of uric acid), and even by stress.

You can easily check the level of the acidity in your body: Get acidity strips (PH-measurement strips can be purchased cheaply at every pharmacy), and test your saliva and your urine. If they are not normal (PH-measurement 7) but acidic (the measurement is lower than 6), then the best thing for you to do would be to have all your amalgam fillings removed immediately. Measure your saliva several times a day, because certain meals might influence the acid level of your saliva. The most reliable test for acidity is that of the first urine of the day.

Medications That Weigh Us Down

Normally, if we take a certain medication for a couple of days, it should not cause too much damage to our systems. A good example of this is the type of medication commonly taken during colds in order to reduce the fever. However, this is not the case with antibiotics. Within just a few days of taking antibiotics, the intestinal flora (see page 15) is damaged to such a degree that a long period of immune deficiency in the intestines is sure to follow. This might also lead to frequent infections.

Every medication that is taken for an extended period of time over several years or even months will cause damage to the liver and the kidneys, which are the organs responsible for cleansing the body of poisons. The medications that are highlighted in the box are especially damaging.

If you already have problems with your liver, gallbladder, or kidneys, and are taking medications, you should be particularly careful. If these organs are already sick, their ability to break down or excrete the medications is limited. For this reason, within one week you might get a triple dose of the active ingredient of the medication, in comparison to the original dose that you planned on having in your system. If this becomes the case, you will not be able to avoid the possible side effects that are mentioned in the brochure that comes with the medication.

Danger from Medications

❖ Blood pressure medications (such as ACE inhibitors and beta blockers)
❖ Heart medications (such as nifedipine preparations)
❖ Cures for rheumatism (infection-blocking medications, Voltan)
❖ Painkillers (including over-the-counter varieties)
❖ Psychiatric drugs
❖ Medications that contain cortisone
❖ Cancer-restraining medications
❖ Immune-suppressive medications

Chronic Disease Syndrome

Some chronic illnesses are accompanied by chronic fatigue. To avoid getting to the point where you are living in complete unawareness of such a disease, your doctor should check for symptoms periodically.

Typical: Diabetes, anemia, chronic intestinal diseases, chronic lung diseases, chronic heart diseases, sleep apnea, serious arteriosclerosis

Diabetes Mellitus (Blood-Sugar Disease)

There are millions of people worldwide who suffer from this metabolic disease. The disease is usually caused by the pancreas not producing enough of the insulin hormone. In many cases, this disease is inherited.

There are two types of diabetes:

❖ Diabetes type 1 is usually found in young people and can be controlled by daily injections of insulin.

❖ Diabetes type 2 is also referred to as "old-age diabetes." It afflicts people who are in their forties and sometimes even people in their sixties. It is possible to treat this type of diabetes through a sugar-free diet and the regular administration of tablets. It is rare that this type of diabetes will require insulin injections.

Constant tiredness can be a symptom of the preliminary stage of diabetes, so this should be regarded as an alarm signal. You can get sugar-test stubs or strips from your pharmacy or doctor that will enable you to check your morning urine for traces of sugar in a relatively convenient manner. However, these tests will give you only a general idea of your overall condition. For a diagnosis that is medically more accurate, further tests are necessary.

Anemia (Blood Deficiency)

The red color of the blood corpuscles comes from the substance hemoglobin (Hb), which contains iron and gives the blood its distinctive color. In the lungs, every blood corpuscle binds oxygen to its blood color and transports it to cells within the body (see drawing on page 30). When there is a lack of red blood color, red blood corpuscles (erythrosines), or iron, this results in anemia, a condition in which none of the organs are supplied with enough oxygen. When people are anemic, their physical and mental performance levels are lowered. The following are possible causes of anemia:

❖ Lack of iron in the primary sources of nutrition

❖ Lack of vitamin B-12

❖ Lack of folic acid (a type of B-complex vitamin)

❖ The beginnings of a liver disease, which can lead to an impairment of the body's ability to take in iron and vitamins

❖ Extensive loss of blood during menstruation, result-

Tip

▼

The self-test is recommended in the case of older people. If diabetes is not recognized for many years and thus goes untreated, it can cause serious eye damage that cannot be corrected with glasses.

Important

If you are noticeably pale or have a strong tendency to get black-and-blue marks, then you may need to seek treatment from a doctor.

ing from a hormonal dysfunction or a clotting disorder (the blood is too thin and flows too quickly)

❖ Clotting disorder, resulting from a liver problem caused by a vitamin-K deficiency, so there is a tendency to develop black-and-blue marks or have bleeding gums (this is observed more in women than in men and may well be the result of taking birth-control pills)

❖ Rare diseases of the bone marrow

A tendency to develop black-and-blue marks and bleeding of the gums: These might be signs of a vitamin-K deficiency.

Chronic Intestinal Diseases

Chronic diarrhea-related diseases, such as an infection of the small intestine (Crohn's disease) and an infection of the large intestine (ulcerative colitis), are fairly rare and seldom remain undiscovered. Frequent diarrhea (up to ten times a day) forces the patient to seek medical help. The doctor can make a diagnosis by conducting a few intestinal tests and taking samples of intestinal mucus.

Chronic Lung Diseases

In cases of chronic bronchitis, chronic or allergic asthma, or emphysema (dilated air spaces in the lungs), the lungs are unable to lead enough oxygen into the blood, causing the entire body to suffer from a chronic oxygen deficiency. People who suffer from this deficiency always fight for air after every minor effort, have to stop to catch their breath several times while climbing stairs, and often have large blown-up chests. If you have any of these symptoms and are not in treatment, you should see a lung specialist (a pulmonary specialist) right away.

Chronic Heart Problems

In the case of chronic heart problems, there is also an oxygen deficiency in the body. In this case, the lungs transport enough oxygen to the blood but the heart is unable to carry the oxygen any further. This inability can have various causes:

❖ Chronic weakness of the heart muscle (an insufficiency in the heart)

❖ Narrowed coronary blood vessels, as the result of arteriosclerosis (angina pectoris)

❖ Preliminary stage of a heart attack ❖ Defects in the valves of the heart

Important

The most common complaints associated with heart diseases (breathing difficulties, swollen legs, frequent urination during the night) are felt relatively late; therefore, if you have any of these symptoms, you should see a heart doctor (a cardiologist) immediately.

Important

If you have apnea, you should inform your doctor about it right away. Apnea can cause complicated and dangerous problems, such as high blood pressure, cardiac dysrhythmia, heart attacks, and strokes.

Apnea (Transient Cessation of Respiration during Sleep)

The milder form of this sleeping disorder is simply referred to as snoring. However, in the typical form, breathing during sleep often ceases for ten seconds or more and then returns with an explosive snoring sound. Although those with apnea do not realize that anything different has taken place, their partners usually wake up from the sound and begin to fear for the lives of their loved ones. Apnea mostly effects men, especially men who are overweight and forty-five years of age or older. Due to the constant interruptions in their sleep, people who suffer from apnea are usually tired during the day and on edge and have difficulties concentrating.

Arteriosclerosis (Vascular Calcification in Older People)

The blood is enriched with oxygen in the pulmonary alveolus and transports the oxygen through the blood vessels (arteries) to the cells of all the organs.

A calcification of the blood vessels can be the reason why an insufficient amount of oxygen reaches the brain and the various vital organs. This can lead to failure symptoms, including forgetfulness, concentration difficulties, and sleeping problems. In time, it can also result in the development of chronic fatigue.

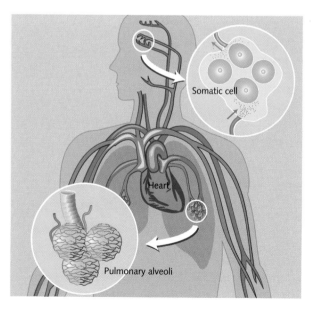

Somatic cell

Heart

Pulmonary alveoli

Chronic Fatigue Syndrome

Chronic fatigue syndrome (CFS) is the only form of fatigue that is accepted by conventional medicine as a disease. In order to verify the disease, certain conditions have to be met and various physical and psychological causes of other diseases have to be ruled out (see page 93).

It is my opinion that the term "chronic fatigue syndrome" serves as a general name for a wide variety of unexplainable fatigue syndromes. In my many years of practice, I have never come across a single patient whose syndromes could be diagnosed solely in accordance with CFS. Nevertheless, I would like to introduce you to the symptoms of this disease. In order to diagnose CFS, at least two of the principal criteria and from six to eight of the secondary criteria need to be met.

The Principal Criteria

❖ Extreme exhaustion that lasts for a period of at least six consecutive months, that does not go away after resting in bed, sleeping, or going on vacation, and that wasn't so severe in the past

❖ A reduction in the usual daily performance level by at least 50 percent

❖ The ruling out of the possibility of any other physical or mental illness, as determined by a standard medical examination (see page 93)

Typical: Two of the primary criteria and at least six to eight of the secondary criteria must be met. All other physical and mental disorders must be ruled out.

The Secondary Criteria

❖ Slight increase in the average body temperature, between 99.5 and 101.5° F (37.5° and 38.6° C)

❖ Shivering

❖ Sore throat

❖ Constantly swollen and eventually painful lymph nodes in the armpits or the throat

❖ Unexplainable weakness of the muscles or muscular pain

❖ Strenuous activities followed by twenty-four hours of fatigue

❖ Irregular headaches

❖ Nerve dysfunction and failure symptoms, such as extreme sensitivity to light or temporary failure of sight (facial failure symptoms)

❖ Mental symptoms, such as forgetfulness, depressive moods, excessive excitement, confusion, concentration difficulties, or orientation problems

❖ Increased need for sleep or recurring difficulty in falling asleep and sleeping through the night appearing consistently over a period of several months

❖ Sudden appearance and disappearance of these symptoms—within a matter of a few days

What Type of Fatigue Do You Have?

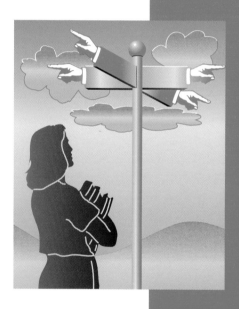

In this chapter, you will find out
which type of fatigue you suffer
from by taking a simple self-test.
You will learn how to distinguish
between the various forms of
fatigue, in order to arrive at a clear
diagnosis. You will also discover
what kinds of therapy are available
to you and what you can do yourself to improve your health.

How to Recognize Your Type of Fatigue

Looking for advice on the subject of fatigue is like standing at a crossroads with ten different signposts. You have a general idea as to where the various roads go but are not sure which road is the right one for you. In order to be able to discern which advice to follow, I suggest that you take the self-test offered here (page 34). Please observe the warning (Important Note on page 96) in the event that you suffer from acute symptoms.

A Note before You Begin

It's important to answer the questions in the test truthfully, for it is only then that this short list of questions can lead you along the right path. Check off all the questions in the test to which you can answer "yes."

Evaluation

The questions are evaluated in groups of four. Every group of four questions to which you answered "yes three or four times leads you to your own type of fatigue. Sometimes this might even be more than one type (a mixed type). In this case, you should read the information on each one of the different types. If this self-test does not give you a clear idea of which form(s) of fatigue you have, it would be best to schedule an appointment with a doctor for a more complete and detailed test.

Evaluation Table

You have answered the following questions with a "yes" more than twice	Your fatigue type	Pages for further reading
1–4	Depressive disorder syndrome	Page 35
5–8	Overtaxed nerves syndrome	Page 37
9–12	Immune deficiency syndrome	Page 40
13–16	Circulatory disorder syndrome	Page 41
17–20	Hormone imbalance syndrome	Page 43
21–24	Metabolic disorder syndrome	Page 45
25–28	Malnutrition syndrome	Page 47
29–32	Poison and allergy syndromes	Page 49
33–36	Chronic disease syndrome	Page 51
37–40	Chronic fatigue syndrome	Page 53

Self-Test: Which Fatigue Category Do You Fit Into?

No.	Question	Yes?
1	Do you lack hope and perspective regarding the future?	❑
2	Have you ever thought of committing suicide?	❑
3	Did you recently take care of a family member for an extended period of time?	❑
4	Has anyone close to you died over the last couple of years?	❑
5	Do you sleep badly and not feel well rested afterward?	❑
6	Do you often suffer from pains in the neck and back due to tight muscles?	❑
7	Do you suffer from fear when you are in close spaces, like an elevator, or do you have a fear of being alone?	❑
8	Are you under a lot of pressure at home or at work?	❑
9	Do you have colds three or more times a year?	❑
10	Is your well-being influenced by the weather?	❑
11	Do you often have herpes lip blisters?	❑
12	Do you work in an air-conditioned environment?	❑
13	Do you have to get out of bed slowly so that you won't get dizzy, or do you get dizzy after bending down?	❑
14	Do you feel especially tired in the morning?	❑
15	Is your nose stuffed during the night? Are you hoarse or do you have excessive mucus in the morning?	❑
16	Do you get headaches when the weather changes or when there is a strong wind?	❑
17	Were you recently pregnant or breast-feeding?	❑
18	Did you feel soreness in your breasts in connection with the above?	❑
19	Are you often extremely sensitive, and do you cry easily?	❑
20	Are you suffering from hot flashes during menopause?	❑
21	Do you often get flatulence, constipation, stomach cramps, or diarrhea?	❑
22	Do you frequently wake up between 1 and 3 A.M.?	❑
23	After lunch, are you tired and do you need to take a nap?	❑
24	Is drinking two glasses of wine or two bottles of beer more than you can handle?	❑
25	Do you tend to get black-and-blue marks from minor injuries?	❑
26	Do you have an intestinal fungus?	❑
27	Do you tend to get cramps in your calves, or are you very pale?	❑
28	Do you eat fast food more than three times a week?	❑
29	Do you take medications for asthma, blood pressure, heart ailments, or psychological problems?	❑
30	Do you have eczema, neurodermatitis, or any food allergies?	❑
31	Is there wood in your home that was treated with varnish before 1986?	❑
32	Are you exposed to solvents, exhaust fumes, or environmental poisons?	❑
33	Have you recently gotten over a long sickness or had shingles?	❑
34	Do you have diabetes?	❑
35	Do you suffer from high blood pressure (especially in the lower values)?	❑
36	Did you ever have a form of cancer?	❑
37	Do you have a fever of around 100.4 degrees F (38 degrees C) while moving around but not while lying in bed?	❑
38	Are the lymph nodes in your throat swollen?	❑
39	Do you still feel tired even after sleeping for eleven hours or more?	❑
40	Do you suffer from unexplained muscular weakness or pain?	❑

Advice for Combating Depressive Disorders

Your type of fatigue is referred to as "depressive disorder syndrome" (see page 11) if depressive moods, along with exhaustion, are a central theme in your life.

Depression as a Reaction to External Events

The process of grieving over the loss of a loved one requires time—sometimes more than a year—and cannot be influenced to much of an extent. However, it may be helpful to speak with someone whom you trust and you know is a good listener and has also experienced a similar loss at some point in his or her life. If you don't have such a friend, or if you find that you have lost the desire to go on living, then it would be a good idea to get some professional help.

Talking with an appropriate person

   Whether you are grieving over the loss of a loved one or are depressed over another external event, members of the clergy, psychologists, workers at suicide centers, and operators of suicide hot lines can help you find the courage to go on living and discover a new purpose in life.

Depression with an Inner Cause

When there are no external causes that can explain your depression, the possibility of your suffering from some physical ailment must be considered. In this case,

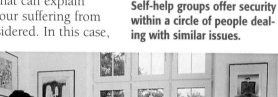

Self-help groups offer security within a circle of people dealing with similar issues.

it is important to get a clear overview of the entire situation and to rule out certain diseases. Ask your family doctor for referrals to colleagues who can check for thyroid diseases and metabolic disorders (an internist), nerve ailments and brain diseases (a neurologist), and hormonal disorders (in the case of a female, a gynecologist).

   If you do not get any clear results from these examinations, I would recommend that

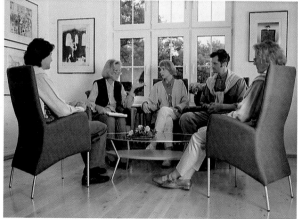

you carry out a special test based on natural medicine (naturopathy), such as a thermoregulation diagnosis (see page 56), a BEV test (see page 57), or a bio-dynamic protein test (see page 56). These tests can often reveal a hidden liver-related depression (see page 12).

Special Case: Liver Disease

Medications worsen the complaints.

In the case of a liver disease, every conventional (chemical) medicine will actually worsen your situation, because the already weakened liver is forced to break down the medication even though it is designed to improve your condition. You should definitely check for the three contagious liver viruses: hepatitis A, B, and C. Earlier liver diseases can flare up with heavy symptoms. But not all liver diseases are caused by bacteria, viruses, or fungi. Chronic stress, such as repressed anger, can bring about the same results.

Appropriate Therapies

❖ Suicidal tendencies brought on by depression can be the result of a problem in the metabolic system. Homeopathy can help in such cases (see page 71).
❖ The movement therapy of Dr. Trager (see page 62) releases emotional tension.
❖ A homeopathic doctor can select specific homeopathic remedies to treat your depression.
❖ The Norwegian success with UV rays (UV-B and UV-C, page 60) has led to this therapy for treating depression being offered in other countries as well.
❖ You can read about the available therapies for hormonal imbalance during menopause on page 44.
❖ There are a number treatments for liver problems that vary according to the specific condition: detoxification or fasting cures, increased doses of vitamin B (see page 69), infusions of your own blood with ozone (see page 58), and homeopathic detoxification.

What You Can Do Yourself

Help with starting the day

A common reaction to the various depressive disorders is a lack of motivation in getting out of bed in the morning. If you have trouble rising in the morning on your own, ask a family member or a roommate to prod you a little.

❖ Kneipp, the priest who rediscovered water treatment, recommends taking a shower right after waking up (see page 85).
❖ Every kind of athletic activity designed to increase stamina (see page 81) is good for counteracting depression and lethargy. Joining a gym or a group of people who play sports together would be ideal and would also increase your motivation.
❖ Herbal remedies, such as Saint-John's-wort capsules, are helpful in combating depressive disorders (see page 88).

Helpful Hints for Relieving Overtaxed Nerves

If stress, along with burnout, is the major issue in your life, you may be suffering from what is referred to as "overtaxed nerves syndrome" (see page 13). You may be overtaxed as a result of not being able to rest because something is continually keeping you in motion. This "something" may have to do with a desire to get attention, be accepted, and gain external recognition. As a result, you take too many tasks upon yourself, and this in turn leads to chronic signs of burnout. There can be various motives for undertaking too much, and attempts at explaining them are found in everything from modern psychology to the ancient system of the anagram, which recognizes nine different personality types in the search for recognition:
❖ **Perfectionists** overtax themselves, because they want to give everything 150 percent. They draw their reassurance from the appreciation that they receive for their work.
❖ **Helpers** sacrifice themselves for the people around them, and as a result they are continuously overtaxed. They don't respect their own physical, mental, and emotional borders, and therefore tend to suffer from chronic disorders (such as gallstones).
❖ **Managers** are addicted to working for success, which provides them with their external image. They treat their own bodies as success machines without any borders.
❖ **Artists** tend to play a new role every day, and they need to devote a lot of time to the staging of these roles. However, the recognition that they seek has to do with making every day turn out to be something special.

Nine personality types reflecting different means of motivation

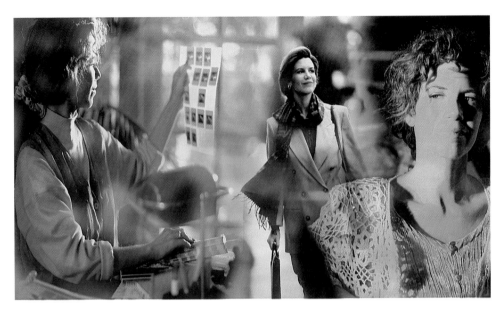

Dreamers want all of their ideas to be realized without delay.

❖ **Thinkers** are rarely overtaxed, because they devote a lot of time to their mental and spiritual worlds, and therefore have a solid self-defense.

❖ **Consistent individuals** are devoted to their points of view and their regular activities "until death do us part." They work in spite of illness and gain approval through their daily reliability.

❖ **Dreamers** indulge themselves every day in a new idea that they would like to realize immediately if possible. For this reason, they have no peace of mind.

❖ **Macho types** constantly try to conquer their surroundings, and they live according to the assumption that an attack is the best defense—even when no one wants to attack them! This stance in life costs them a lot of energy.

❖ **Pacifists** tend to have such a fear of confrontation that they end up turning all their aggressions against themselves. They often appear to be inactive and lazy. Their stress is revealed only internally.

Try to let go of a compulsive need for approval.

Regardless of what category you fit into, take the alarm signals that your body is sending you seriously and try to free yourself from a compulsive need for approval. Think about whether or not you would benefit from therapy. Change your lifestyle before something like a heart attack changes it for you.

Appropriate Therapies

❖ The movement therapy of Dr. Trager (see page 62) releases physical and mental tension related to stress.
❖ Manual muscle therapy (see page 63) releases painful muscular tension.
❖ Shiatsu massage (see page 61) harmonizes the energy of the body.
❖ Continuous shower therapy (see page 65) is one of the fastest ways to release stress.

What You Can Do Yourself

❖ Plan your daily schedule: Take out fifteen minutes a day for this purpose on a regular basis. This time will give you a better perspective and release you from the hectic pace of everyday life.
❖ Give yourself some time to do what you enjoy: If you are an intellectual type of person, reserve some time for reading. If you are athletic, make some time for sports. If you are creative, set aside some time for artistic activities.
❖ Be conscious of not releasing your nervousness on the people around you. Instead, try participating in competitive sports, and don't forget about the social aspect that comes with these activities.
❖ Create some space for yourself in order to be able to

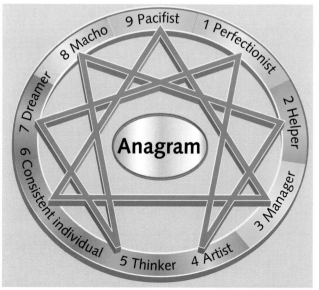

The nine personality types recognized by the anagram

reflect on life. Sometimes this is easier to do in a group than alone. Consider taking a course in meditation (see page 79), yoga, or religious or spiritual practices, or doing any other type of group activity that allows you to think of larger issues or still your mind.

❖ Learn about relaxation techniques that resonate with you.

❖ Take advantage of anti-stress seminars.

❖ Herbs, such as valerian and kava kava, are relaxing in cases of anxiety.

Measures for Overcoming Immune Deficiency

If you are always tired and frequently get infections, you may be suffering from a type of fatigue known as "immune deficiency syndrome."

A Collapse of the Immune System Due to Stress

Why people sometimes get sick while on vacation

Stress puts the body into a constant state of alarm, which also stimulates the immune system. When this constant stimulation ceases (for example, when you go on vacation), then the immune system often collapses. Your body takes the longest possible time to detoxify itself—an activity that it never previously had time for—and releases waste products in a number of different ways, such as developing infected tonsils or feverish sweating. This situation can be cured by a long-lasting stress release (see pages 39).

Disorders of the Intestinal Flora (from Taking Antibiotics)

Disorders of the intestinal flora may lead to a serious immune-deficiency condition accompanied by the growth of rotting bacteria and fungi (see page 15). In this case, infections in the throat and bronchial area often develop. For signs of a fungus attack, see page 16.

Appropriate Therapies

❖ Have your family doctor take a blood test or an intestinal test to check for fungi. To determine the condition of your immune system, there are two naturopathic tests you should consider taking: the candida immune profile test and the immune skin test (see page 57).

❖ In order to build up your intestinal flora, you should take certain combinations of bacteria cultures for a period of six to twelve months. This is a must after taking antibiotics.

❖ In the case of mild disorders of the intestinal flora, a form of colon hydrotherapy (or enema) can be helpful in relieving the immune system (see page 67). In more complicated cases, a form of symbiotic influence may be necessary (see page 68). This treatment requires patience, as it can last from one to two years, although its positive effects can already be felt after a few months.

Enemas are purifying and regenerating.

What You Can Do Yourself

❖ Release your stress with helpful meditation exercises (see page 79).

❖ Strengthen your immune system by taking an alternating warm-and-cold shower on a daily basis (see page 85), exercising regularly (see page 81), and paying a weekly visit to the sauna (see page 85).

❖ Reduce your consumption of sweets drastically. My personal recommendation is as follows: Eat sweets only after a full meal, not in between meals, and not in addition to the main course. Concentrated sugar can be very damaging to the maintenance of healthy intestinal flora if it is consumed on an empty stomach.

❖ If you want to avoid suffering a collapse of the immune system during your vacation, then you might consider undergoing a short-term therapy (about two weeks prior to your vacation) entailing taking a variety of herbal remedies designed to enhance the immune system (see page 87).

The valves of the veins are responsible for not allowing the blood to flow backward. In the case of widened veins (varicose veins), the valves do not close completely.

Suggestions for Dealing with Circulatory Disorders

If you suffer from a circulatory ailment, along with fatigue, you may have what is referred to as "circulatory disorder syndrome" (see page 17). Blood pressure values that differ from the norm do not necessarily indicate the presence of problems, as it all depends on which category you fall into. The body could get adjusted to the condition and not show any signs of a problem. However, if you truly suffer from a circulatory ailment (see page 17), you should be examined by your family doctor. Special cases of circulatory disorders are as follows:

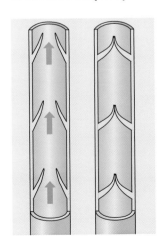

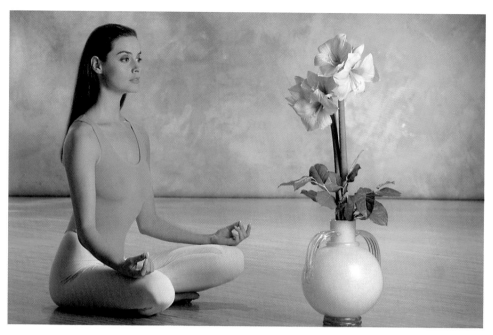

Through deep relaxation in meditation, you can reach an inner state of balance, which has a healing effect in every case of burnout.

Varicose Veins

After giving birth several times, women often suffer from varicose veins. The widening of the veins makes it harder for the blood to travel back to the heart. The blood accumulates in the legs, and the lymphatic fluids from the blood make the legs swollen.

Cold Hands and Feet

If your hands and feet are constantly freezing, you might be suffering from a chronic circulatory disorder. With people who are younger than fifty years of age, this could be the result of a liver disorder or poisoning from a wood varnish, which leads to tension in the muscles connected to the blood vessels.

Appropriate Therapies

❖ If you suffer from varicose veins, you should consult a specialist. However, it's important to be aware that operating on the veins will not be the ultimate solution, because this will cause the remaining veins to wear out faster. There is no ultimate solution for this condition, but you can improve the situation by exercising the musculature supporting the blood vessels through the regular use of a variety of water therapies (see page 83).

❖ In the case of swollen legs, lymphatic drainage (see page 66) and continuous shower therapy (see page 65) can be very effective.

❖ In extreme cases of circulatory weakness, you can get herbal supplements from your doctor, and they do not have any side effects. But just as is the case with conventional remedies, the herbal remedies also do not necessarily guarantee that the condition will be healed.

❖ Ozone therapy (see page 58) and the oxygen inhalation therapy of Professor Ardenne (see page 60) bring long-lasting improvement for those who suffer from cold hands and feet.

What You Can Do Yourself

❖ Gingko leaves in the form of a tea or as a remedy are helpful in treating cold hands and feet.

❖ Give your circulation a healthy workout by taking a refreshing warm-and-cold shower (see page 85) every morning and by regularly performing exercises designed to increase your physical stamina (see page 81). Fifteen minutes of exercise every morning, on a regular basis, will definitely bolster your circulation.

❖ Flower pollens (see page 92) also accelerate the circulation in a harmless manner.

Recommendations for Regulating Hormonal Imbalances

You may be suffering from a type of fatigue known as "hormonal imbalance syndrome" (see page 19) if depressive moods, along with fatigue, are a major issue in your life.

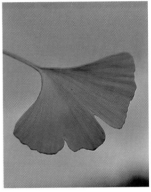

The leaf of the gingko, an ancient tree of eastern China

Female Hormonal Disorders during Youth

If your periods are very irregular and you suffer from severe cramps, you should try to discover the cause of these problems (it's possible that you have an infection in your ovaries or a thyroid disorder). In cases of hormonal disorders accompanied by soreness in the breasts before one's period, a tendency to develop cysts in the ovaries, or severe menstrual cramps, the only assistance available may come from the diagnostic procedures of naturopathy, such as thermoregulation diagnosis and the bio-dynamic protein profile (see page 56).

Hormonal Disorders during and after Menopause

Look for hidden causes.

Even though menopause—which is influenced by one's genes—can set in before the age of fifty-two without implying any problems, it's always a good idea in cases of an early onset to be checked for a hormonal disorder, which might take the form of a hidden ovary infection. Because regular gynecological tests can reveal an infection only in its acute state, I would recommend the thermoregulation diagnosis or a bio-dynamic protein test (see page 56). In cases of acute hormone deficiency symptoms, your gynecologist should take a blood test.

Thyroid Disorders

A goiter is an enlargement of the thyroid gland that is often due to a nutrition-related iodine deficiency (see page 19). But it can also appear in girls during puberty as a result of an ovary infection that is caused by their being exposed to below-normal temperatures. Through the interaction of the various hormone glands, this situation can lead to a hyperfunctioning of the thyroid gland.

Adrenaline Deficiency of the Suprarenal Gland

Adrenaline is a hormone that is released in the body in situations of stress (and fear). Dogs and other animals can smell this hormone. The bio-dynamic blood test (see page 56) can detect slight adrenaline deficiency symptoms. This rare disorder has to be treated by a specialist (an endocrinologist).

Appropriate Therapies

❖ Single or complex homeopathic remedies (see page 71) can be helpful in cases of hormone disorders accompanied by soreness in the breasts. Conventional hormone medications cannot help in such cases.
❖ Homeopathy (see page 71) and enzyme therapy (see page 91) are helpful in treating chronic ovary infections. You should be aware of the fact that a diagnostic examination using ultrasound at a gynecologist's office will generally not reveal such infections.

What You Can Do Yourself

❖ If you suffer from problems related to menopause, you can activate your self-healing powers in the following four ways:
❖ Water therapy (see page 83) on a regular basis. For

Warning

When discontinuing a treatment with hormone tablets or patches, it is not uncommon for a woman to suffer from various infections and severe hot flashes for several months.

example, twice a week take a twenty-minute bath with chamomile extract added to the water, followed by thirty minutes of relaxation in bed.

❖ Aerobic exercise (see page 81).

❖ Maintaining a steady diet of whole foods, primarily consisting of vegetarian foods—this is important for your overall well-being. Eliminate salt from your diet as much as you can to prevent fluids from accumulating in your tissue. Your diet should be low in fat and carbohydrates but high in proteins. Stay away from alcohol, coffee, and nicotine. Do your best to lose any excess weight. Losing weight can, by itself, regulate many of the problems associated with menopause.

❖ Herbal remedies, such as black cohosh (see page 90) and Saint-John's-wort (see page 88).

❖ If you have an iodine deficiency, eat food rich in iodine (such as iodized sea salt and fish from the sea) or take iodine in the form of a medication. Go on regular vacations to the beach, where you can breathe the fresh sea air that is rich in iodine and eat ocean fish.

❖ If you discontinue a hormone tablet or hormone patch treatment, it can be helpful to use homeopathic herbal remedies that are similar to hormones (such as rhubarb extract) and/or biological medications (such as spleen extract); take two capsules once a day over a period of six to twelve months.

❖ If a particular situation is becoming too stressful for you and wearing you down, adenosine (see page 91) can be helpful in enhancing your energy level.

How to Deal with Metabolic Disorders

If problems with your digestive system, along with fatigue, are primary issues in your life, you may be suffering from a type of fatigue known as "metabolic disorder syndrome" (see page 20).

Chronic Liver Disorders

There are only a few liver diseases that are caused by alcohol, but any damaged liver will not be able to tolerate alcohol. The liver is the only organ in the body that can break down alcohol. Therefore, if you got good results on your liver test but still have difficulties tolerating alcohol (see page 20), it is advised to perform a

Tips

If your hot flashes are becoming more severe, put your hands under cold running water. A warm bath with valerian or rosemary bath essence will relax you and help you get a good night's sleep.

What does alcohol intolerance mean?

thermoregulation diagnosis (see page 56) and a BEV test (see page 57) and have bio-dynamic blood work done (see page 56), to determine the actual state of your liver metabolism.

Gallbladder Problems

The typical signs of impaired gallbladder metabolism include a regular need to pass wind (often foul-smelling) or intestinal rumbling, light-colored or even white stools (in such a case, seek medical attention immediately!), frequent diarrhea after eating fatty foods, and very painful gall colic.

In the case of gall problems, the liver must be examined as well.

With the sudden appearance of colic, it's advised to undergo a diagnostic examination using ultrasound to check for gallstones, which can be easily removed with a laser or through a relatively minor operation. However, the matter may be a little more complicated, because all gall problems actually originate from many years of suffering with liver disorders (see page 20). Therefore, it's important to check well in advance for any liver problems.

Chronic Pancreatic Problems

An acute infection of the pancreas usually causes severe cramps. If a chronic infection runs its course without cramps, you may feel a heavy tiredness after every meal.

Chronic Constipation

When constipation lasts several days, waste products stay in the digestive system for the same amount of time. Instead of being released from the system, the retained waste products and poisons begin to burden the metabolic system. A result of this situation can be chronic tiredness and a lack of motivation.

Appropriate Therapies

❖ For liver disorders, there is a long-lasting homeopathic treatment (see page 71).
❖ In the case of a pancreas deficiency, in a medical procedure the doctor is able to replace the missing digestive gastric juices in an artificial way (from a pig's pancreas).
❖ A helpful remedy for chronic constipation is the colon hydrotherapy treatment (see page 67). This treatment can ease the pain and stimulate intestinal movement.

What You Can Do Yourself

❖ In the case of a liver disorder, milk thistle capsules may be helpful (see page 89).

❖ For problems with flatulence, there are several gall teas that you can buy at drugstores or health food stores that will accelerate the functioning of the gallbladder. In addition, garlic (see page 89) and artichoke juice (see page 88) can be helpful.

❖ With every metabolic disorder, it is important to maintain a low-fat diet. Also, you should not eat any fresh fruits or vegetables after 7 P.M. The reason for this is that the liver produces fewer gastric juices at this time, which results in a process of fermentation that will cause you to sleep poorly and restlessly.

❖ If you suffer from constipation, herbal laxative teas can be helpful. Eating bran, taking alfalfa tablets (eight to twelve tablets twice a day), and walking will also help regulate your bowel movements.

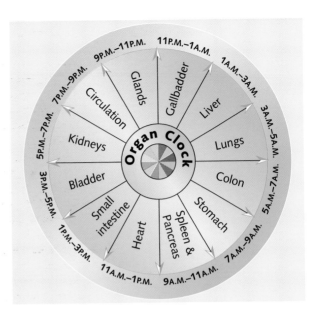

If you always feel bad at the same time, the organ clock might be able to help you discover which of your organs is sick.

According to the organ clock used in acupuncture (see illustration), the intestines are especially active between 5 and 7 A.M. For this reason, the best time for a bowel movement is at the end of this period of activity, at 7 A.M.

Many people find the stimulating effect of coffee, black tea, or green tea helpful (remember not to leave the teabag in the water for more than three minutes). There are only a few gall and digestive diseases that make one unable to tolerate these drinks.

It is essential to your health that you have a bowel movement on a daily basis. If the methods that are recommended above are of no help to you, consult your doctor some stronger herbal remedies.

Combating Malnutrition

If you have vitamin and mineral deficiencies and are tired all the time, you may have the type of fatigue known as "malnutrition syndrome" (see page 22).

Vitamin Deficiency in Children

Many children simply do not eat enough fruits and vegetables, in spite of their mothers' efforts to convince them to do so and preparing their food for them. Sometimes this is the result of a liver disorder with which the children were born. In such cases, their skin was yellow for a while after their birth. Throughout their childhood, they are very stubborn in refusing to eat any fruits or vegetables because of the stomachache that doing so causes them. The result of this condition is a vitamin deficiency.

Vitamin Deficiency as the Result of Poor Eating Habits

Vitamin deficiency from eating fast food

Elderly people usually eat small portions of food, because they don't move around very much. If, in addition, they get their food from a large kitchen (such as at an old-age home), this can lead over the years to a nutrition-related vitamin deficiency. The working sectors of populations in large cities suffer from the same condition due to the hectic pace of big-city life; many working people eat fast food and meals kept warm over an extended period of time in cafeterias and restaurants (see page 23). Cigarettes, alcohol, and the consumption of sweets cause further deficiencies.

Hypoglycemia (Low Blood Sugar)

If you suffer from this disorder (see page 24), try to stay away from any foods containing sugar (including jams and honey) because they can cause you to feel shaky or nervous. In addition to eating the normal three meals a day, seriously consider eating a snack in the morning and the afternoon.

Appropriate Therapies

❖ In the case of improper nutrition, I would recommend that you seek professional counseling, which would enable you to receive treatment targeted to your specific situation and provide you with the appropriate nutritional supplements (see page 90).

❖ In order to check for the exact deficiencies that you suffer from, your doctor or your homeopathic healer can conduct a vitamin analysis based on your blood work (which is unfortunately very expensive).

❖ In the case of low sugar in the blood, your doctor

should give you a sugar capacity test so that he or she can provide you with precise instructions for your diet. If you suffer from fatigue caused by liver problems, turn to the discussion on page 45.

Healthy nutrition heals all kinds of deficiencies.

What You Can Do Yourself

❖ It might seem futuristic, but try taking chewable fruit and vegetable lozenges. They exist in two forms: higher potency for adults and lower potency for children.
❖ For older people, there are special supplements (which can be obtained at drugstores or from distributors) that contain a mixture of minerals and vitamins designed especially for the needs of this age group. The usual recommended dosage is two capsules in the morning on a daily basis.
❖ Most nutritional deficiencies can be combated by changing your diet and eating healthy foods. In addition to getting assistance from a nutritionist, there are many books on nutrition that can be helpful.
❖ Smoking cigarettes brings about vitamin deficiencies; it also weakens the immune system and causes cancer, in addition to eating up your paycheck. Make a commitment to give it up.
❖ If you drink alcohol on a regular basis, it should not exceed one glass of wine or two glasses of beer (16 fl. oz) a day. Should you end up drinking a lot at a party one night, give your liver at least three to five days to recover, during which time you must not drink any alcohol. Try to even out the deficiency by taking vitamin B-complex (one to two capsules twice a day).
❖ If you have liver problems, note the suggestions on pages 45–46.

After parties, allow your liver time to recover.

Counteracting Poisons and Allergies

You may have an allergy or poison syndrome (see page 24) if you are plagued by allergies or a broad range of unclear symptoms in addition to fatigue.

Unclear complaints in the case of poisoning

Acute Poisoning or Allergies

In the case of acute poisoning or a life-threatening allergy (such as a bee sting in the throat), you must get to the nearest doctor as soon as possible. When a situation is life-threatening, anything that helps you at that moment is the proper solution.

Chronic Poisoning

I have already discussed the various types of poisoning that can take place over the course of a longer period of time and that may occur as the result of exposure to environmental toxins (see page 25). Unfortunately, most of us are not aware of many of these dangers. For example, you might enjoy making stained-glass windows of lead and glass, without ever considering that this seemingly harmless hobby could cause lead poisoning. Therefore, whenever you cannot identify the cause of your symptoms, you should think about the possibility of poisoning. This suspicion, however, must be verified through the appropriate diagnostic methods (see page 55).

Chronic Allergies

The appearance of allergies has increased drastically both in their number and in the progressively dramatic forms that they take. The massive repression of symptoms of illnesses that is carried out by conventional medicine cannot help in the case of allergies. What is recommended is that you search for the cause of your allergy by means of the bio-dynamic blood test (see page 56) and then look for a naturopath who specializes in your type of allergy. In most cases, allergy sufferers can do without cortisone, which causes liver damage and immune deficiency.

Quicksilver Poisoning

If having an overly acidic metabolism causes the quicksilver (mercury) to be released from the amalgam fillings in your teeth and therefore induces poisoning, the only solution is a radical removal of all the amalgam fillings, accompanied by a treatment that helps lead the quicksilver out of the body. Be sure to get information about the materials that will replace your amalgam fillings, because even gold fillings can be made out of poisonous compounds.

Amalgam—the creeping poison

Side Effects of Medications

If you suffer from liver or gall problems, it is likely that they are somehow related to the side effects of medications. This is even possible when the gamma-GT liver value is normal (see page 20). Speak to your doctor about possible natural substitutes for the medications that you are taking right now. If you have doubts regarding your doctor's opinion, consult a naturopath.

Even in the case of antibiotics (see page 27), there are substitutes, such as homeopathic remedies, that do not cause any side effects and can be applied in many cases.

Appropriate Therapies

❖ Detoxifying the body from specific poisons (such as quicksilver) can be carried out by means of applying complex allopathic methods, especially homeopathic remedies (see page 71).
❖ Allergies can be treated in various ways, including taking various minerals, such as calcium, and using homeopathic remedies, symbiotic influence (see page 68), and methods designed to stimulate the immune system, such as infusions of your own blood with ozone (see page 58) and bio-resonance therapy (see page 73).

What You Can Do Yourself

❖ You must remove all the poisonous objects in your house, such as wood paneling that was treated with toxic varnish. If you are not sure whether or not anything is toxic in your home, you can have the toxic level of the air there checked. However, these tests are not always reliable. The best way to obtain a definite answer is by having blood work done, in order to see if any kind of poisoning has entered your system.
❖ Self-treatments against allergies (for example, with hay fever drops) are usually not very effective. If you have allergies related to the seasons, calcium tablets can sometimes help (take one 500 mg tablet per day over the course of three months).

Take a measurement of the toxicity of the air in your home, and have blood work done.

Assistance in the Case of Chronic Diseases

If your complaints are related to a particular disease, in addition to fatigue, you may be suffering from a type of fatigue known as "chronic disease syndrome" (see page 27).

Diabetes

In the case of diabetes, regular medical treatment is indispensable. The disease has a negative influence on all the blood vessels, which is why many circulatory disturbances may appear, first in the more delicate vessels in the eyes and then in the rest of the organs.

Anemia

In this case, you have to be sure of the exact cause of the disease, otherwise the appropriate treatment cannot be administered.

First determine the cause.

Chronic Organ Diseases

Chronic diseases of different organs (see pages 27–30) have to be verified and then treated by a specialist.

Arteriosclerosis (Calcification of the Blood Vessels)

If you experience pronounced forgetfulness, you should have yourself checked for metabolic diseases. Liver diseases and certain poisonings cause similar symptoms. Try not to blame every problem that occurs on your age.

Appropriate Therapies

❖ For diabetes, in addition to the standard insulin treatment, there are naturopathic treatment methods that can help: If you suffer from eye problems, acupuncture (see page 72) can improve many of your difficulties. Homeopathy (see page 71), herbs that stimulate circulation (such as gingko, page 88), ozone treatments (see page 58), and vitamins can be used to treat other symptoms. Moreover, homeopathic remedies can help decrease the amount of insulin that you must take.

❖ In the case of anemia, it is essential to choose the right therapy. Watch out for preparations that contain iron, because they can have a lot of side effects (irritations in the stomach and intestines, buildup of waste products, vomiting, constipation or diarrhea, nervousness, and headaches). Homeopathic remedies can be just as effective in treating anemia.

❖ When it comes to chronic organ diseases, the options for healing the disease with naturopathic remedies depend on the individual case. In general, we can say that it is pos-

Natural medicine as additional therapy

sible to lessen the complaints by combining both natural and conventional medicine, which can also reduce the amount of chemical medication that you must take. If you wish to treat your disease solely with naturopathy, I would recommend that you consult a homeopathic practitioner.

❖ For circulation problems at an advanced age, a vast improvement can be reached through infusions of herbal remedies (see page 87) and ozone therapy (see page 58). These treatments must be repeated on an annual basis.

What You Can Do Yourself

❖ When it comes to a chronic disease, your ability to help yourself is limited to the general rules of leading a healthy life. (See page 76 onward.)

❖ When you want to substitute the conventional medicines that you have been taking with natural healing remedies, you should not quit taking the conventional medicines before consulting your doctor or therapist. In doing this, you could worsen your condition.

Speak with your doctor before you stop using your medications.

What Action You Can Take regarding Chronic Fatigue Syndrome

It is also possible that the type of fatigue that you are suffering from is what is known as "chronic fatigue syndrome" (see page 30). Unfortunately, this type of fatigue cannot be verified solely by the four simple questions in our self-test. In addition to these questions, the criteria that are mentioned on page 31 must be met. If this is the case, then you must prepare yourself to go on a journey through all the different divisions of medicine. First, you have to rule out all the diseases that are mentioned in the appendix (see page 93), which is only possible by submitting to a large number of examinations. Only after you have gone through all of this can you consider your situation as falling under the medical category of "chronic fatigue syndrome."

A journey through the divisions of medicine

Appropriate Therapies

If the medical examinations do not show evidence of the causes of chronic fatigue syndrome, only the symptoms you are experiencing can be treated. For example, a case of apnea, in which the regular flow of breath ceases during the night (usually associated with chronic disease syndrome), can be treated in a sleep laboratory through technical stimulation.

What You Yourself Can Do

❖ There is a special tea blend available at drugstores and health food stores that can be used to combat snoring, which is considered to be a mild form of apnea.

❖ For additional complaints, note the recommendations that are given with regard to the other types of fatigue.

At the Office of the Natural Healing Practitioner

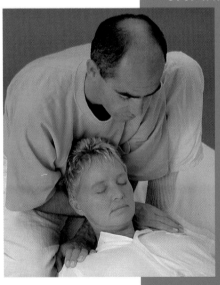

While conventional medicine still argues over whether or not chronic fatigue syndrome (burnout syndrome) should be diagnosed as a disease, and the opinions differ on which cases should actually count as chronic fatigue syndrome, natural medicine offers an abundance of effective diagnostic methods and successful therapies for those who suffer from CFS-like symptoms. In the following chapter, you will learn what these methods and therapies are and how they function.

Photo: Shiatsu, finger-massage therapy

Important Naturopathic Diagnostic Methods

Many of the diagnostic methods of natural medicine (naturopathy) are still not well known, even though they have been proven to lead to the early and exact diagnosis of a number of diseases. It often happens that even the family doctor will not be aware of the presence of these diseases. Therefore, I would like to acquaint you with the most important naturopathic methods for diagnosing chronic fatigue syndrome. This way, you will also be able to request a particular test or examination from your doctor and be able to justify this request in a knowledgeable manner.

Decoder Demography (DD)

In decoder demography, metal plates are placed on the skin. A weak current of electricity flows between the plates and is shown on a measurement apparatus. The individual values are then compared to normal values (that is, they are decoded) and can point to health problems in the assigned organs (see page 72). Many problems that can rarely be diagnosed (and sometimes not be diagnosed at all) by means of conventional methods (see boxes) can be discovered by using this technique. In addition, decoder demography can save you a lot of money on other tests, because it can be used as an objective tool for measuring the progress and effectiveness of your treatment and for getting exact clues regarding further therapy.

Problem Areas in the Body

❖ Bad teeth (due to abscesses, amalgam fillings)
❖ Inflammation of the appendix, gallbladder, ovaries, prostate, or sinuses
❖ Scars, wounds, foreign particles
❖ Encapsulation of what was earlier an infection
❖ Damaged intestinal flora (see page 15)
❖ Deviations of the spine, which cause the nerves to strangulate
❖ Inherited organ weakness or malfunctioning

Other Problem Areas

❖ Physical ailments caused by electromagnetic fields (such as from high-power electric cables or electric cables near your bed), underground water, or contaminated soil
❖ Chemical poisoning, such as from medications or environmental toxins (see pages 25–27)
❖ The effects of a shock or constant psychosomatic disorders (see page 11)
❖ Inability to process basic foods

Advantages of Thermoregulation Diagnosis

❖ Discovering the unknown causes of chronic diseases
❖ Finding the acute or chronic focus of an inflammation, before it can cause long-term health damage
❖ A method of disease prevention for the entire body
❖ Finding weak areas of the organism in generally healthy patients
❖ Helping to monitor a healing process or the results of treatment with a certain medication

Thermoregulation Diagnosis (TRD)

In this procedure, the exact temperature of the entire skin area is measured by means of electrical devices. A computer compares these values with normal values within a few seconds. The result is a temperature pattern that enables your therapist to get a basic idea about the health of your internal organs (see page 72).

The temperature measurement is carried out twice: once before and once after cooling down (usually by means of undressing), which forces the body to regulate its own temperature (thermoregulation). Within a few minutes, every area of the skin tries to adjust to the new temperature.

Some areas of the skin might be cooler than other areas. This means that the circulation is weaker in these areas, which is often the result of an infection in one of the internal organs that is related to this area of the skin. If, on the other hand, we find an increase in the temperature of the skin in a particular area, this is an indication that there is a chronic disease in the related area.

Advantages of the Bio-Dynamic Protein Profile

❖ It often makes intrusive tests, such as punctures and incisions, superfluous.
❖ It often spares you from X rays, contrast media, and computer tomography, and therefore from the effects of radioactivity, allergic reactions, and liver problems.
❖ It is the most accurate type of blood work you can undergo, detecting health problems much earlier than any other method.

Bio-Dynamic Protein Profile

Not only can even the smallest wound, infection, or metabolic disorder cause stress but also a change in the amount, consistency, and electrical charge of proteins in the blood. The bio-dynamic protein profile makes use of this fact in order to diagnose diseases. About 60 units of protein in the blood serum are measured in the laboratory, revealing very exact information concerning the health of the patient. The bio-dynamic protein profile is not only an excellent adjunct to regular blood work, but it can also reveal hidden organ diseases, which conventional blood work cannot do. Furthermore, you can spare yourself a lot of expensive tests and examinations, because this test will show exactly which organ is causing the problem.

Bioelectronics According to Professor Vincent (BEV)

Bioelectronics is a special type of examination that is designed to test the fluids of the body: the blood, saliva, and urine. This test measures, among other things, the following characteristics of the fluids: their acid level (PH-value), their electric resistance, their mineral level, and their state of oxidation. The results of this test show whether or not the organism is healthy and provide information regarding the diseases to which the organism may be susceptible.

Advantages of the Bioelectronic Test

❖ Measures the quality of every fluid (bodily fluids, water, all beverages and dissolved nutrients)
❖ Shows the risk of getting thrombosis, infarcts, cancer (to a limited extent), metabolic diseases, kidney diseases, and lymphatic diseases
❖ Measures the body's immunity against diseases
❖ Reveals the efficiency of different therapies

The Candida Immune Profile

This new method of diagnosing fungal diseases in the blood originated in the United States. The ELISA (Enzyme-Linked Immunosorbent Assay) immune test can measure the cells of the fungus (candida antigen) as well as the proteins that the body produces as immunity against the fungus (candida IgA antibody, candida IgG antibody, and candida IgM antibody). If these particles are present, it means that the body is fighting a fungal infection. The fungus is creating difficulties in the body and requires treatment.

A new method for determining the presence of fungi

The Immune Skin Test

This test measures the reaction of the immune system to seven different substances that are applied to the skin. After forty-eight hours, the results can be read according to the redness of the skin. This test is designed to show how strongly or how weakly the immune system reacts and whether or not it is necessary to undergo a treatment in order to enhance the immune system.

Testing the state of your immune system

Important Naturopathic Therapies

The treatment methods that are mentioned in this book are only a small selection from the vast number of therapies that are available in natural medicine. These methods have proven themselves through years of practice to be very effective in overcoming burnout. In writing about the various methods, I limited myself to describing only the most significant aspects. Therefore, if you are interested in undergoing one of these therapies, I would recommend that you seek more detailed information.

Blood Therapy with Ozone

Ozone is a special form of oxygen in which three oxygen atoms, instead of only two, are combined into one molecule (see drawing on opposite page). Ozone has a tendency to transport the extra oxygen atom to other substances. This quality is the reason why ozone is used medically for the purpose of stimulating the metabolism and the immune system.

Administration of the Therapy

In each therapy session, blood is taken out of the body and mixed with 98 percent oxygen and 2 percent ozone. The blood is then injected back into the body without delay. I have used the following two different kinds of ozone treatment:

A Recommendation for Ozone Therapy

Ozone therapy has been practiced for more than fifty years. It is used worldwide by conventional doctors and practitioners of natural medicine with great success. If administered by an experienced therapist, it is a worthwhile and safe therapy. It is especially effective in the treatment of liver infections (as well as infections caused by viruses) and all sorts of circulatory disorders.

❖ **Small-scale blood treatment.** The therapist takes a full syringe of blood from the vein, mixes it with the ozone-and-oxygen mixture, and injects it back into the gluteal muscle. This procedure is performed twice a week. It is recommended that you undergo at least ten treatments.

❖ **Large-scale blood treatment.** A larger amount of blood is taken. The ozone-and-oxygen mixture is fed into a clear, sterile transfusion bottle. Afterward, the patient receives his or her own blood back into the same vein from which it was originally taken. The advantage of this method is the larger amount of ozone, which has much better results. The improvement ensuing from a cure of ten to twelve infusions (two to three infusions per week) can be felt for an entire year.

Side Effects

If the therapy is done incorrectly, it can lead to excessive sweating, a drop in blood pressure, shock, and embolism.

Areas of Application

❖ Arthritis in all the joints
❖ Hardening of the arteries (pain felt in the area of the heart during physical exertion and while resting)
❖ A variety of liver problems (viruses, alcoholism, infections)
❖ Treatment after a stroke (also for signs of paralysis)
❖ Rheumatic symptoms (for example, muscular rheumatism or joint rheumatism, as well as lumbago and sciatic problems)
❖ An abnormally high level of fat in the blood (cholesterol, triglyceride)
❖ An abnormally high level of uric acid (gout)
❖ Delayed physical recovery from serious diseases, operations, or trauma
❖ Difficult healing of wounds after operations on bones
❖ Recommended as a supplemental therapy for cancer
❖ Useful for all different types of skin disease (such as acne, eczema, psoriasis, dermatitis)
❖ All eye diseases caused by a circulatory problem
❖ Migraine headaches
❖ All kinds of attacks of dizziness
❖ General exhaustion or excessive physical demands

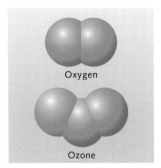

Oxygen

Ozone

The only difference between ozone and oxygen is one additional oxygen atom. A high quantity causes irritations in the eyes and the lungs, whereas a low quantity has a stimulating effect on the metabolic system and the immune system.

Serves a number of purposes

Professor Ardenne's Method of Oxygen Inhalation

There is a saying that "oxygen is life." We gain energy through the burning processes that take place in nutrients and oxygen in every cell of our bodies. If there is a lack of oxygen, there will also be a lack of energy: The organs cannot accomplish their tasks, and you find yourself in a state of exhaustion. Professor Ardenne developed the oxygen inhalation method as a therapy for problems that are caused by an oxygen deficiency. With this method, oxygen is artificially supplied to the sick tissue, in order to enable it to resume its normal activities until it is capable of becoming independent and providing itself with the necessary amount of oxygen.

Administration of the Therapy

Oxygen (out of an oxygen bottle) is mixed with negatively charged ions (see page 65) and then inhaled in this form. The treatment is repeated daily for a period of fifteen to twenty days.

Side Effects

There are no known side effects.

Areas of Application

❖ Lung, heart, and blood diseases
❖ A deficiency of red blood corpuscles (for example, in the case of an iron or vitamin deficiency)
❖ Infections that require more oxygen
❖ Circulatory problems, as the result of arteriosclerosis, for example

Treatment with Ultraviolet Light (UV-B and UV-C)

Known for ages

The healing powers of UV-B and UV-C rays have been known for a long time. They penetrate deep under the skin and stimulate the healing process. In earlier times only tuberculosis patients sought out this therapy, but today anyone suffering from psoriasis can go to the Red Sea where the sunlight there contains almost entirely UV-B and UV-C rays. By contrast, the sunlight in most other places contains mainly UV-A rays. This enables you to tan, but can also result in sunburn and other damaging effects on your skin and your overall health.

Therapy with UV-B and UV-C rays has the following effects:

❖ It increases the skin temperature by 3.5 to 4.5 degrees and has the ability to provide a high level of tissue purification, which results in improved circulation.
❖ Light-sensitive structures in the skin are stimulated by the light and the increased temperature. They initiate a healing process, examples of which can be observed in cases of psoriasis or dermatitis.

Administration of the Therapy

While you are lying down and relaxing, modern radiation devices illuminate your body for twenty to forty minutes with the same amount of light that you would get in the tropics during an entire day.

Side Effects

If you have very light or sensitive skin, you might see a slight reddening of the skin, similar to sunburn. If you have an allergy to the sun, this form of therapy is not advised for you.

Areas of Application

❖ Improved circulation, detoxification, and excretion, as a result of the stimulation of the organs in question
❖ Stimulation of the nervous system as well as the various glands
❖ Stabilization of the acidic protective layer of the skin, which in turn strengthens the body's immune system

Shiatsu Therapy

Shiatsu means "finger pressure." It is a Japanese therapeutic massage that came into existence somewhere around 530 B.C. This method of healing through touch is based on the system of the meridians, which was developed in acupuncture (see page 72). Special techniques of pulling, holding, or shifting the weight of the body stimulate the flow of energy and improve the circulation of the blood and the lymphatic fluids. With

A Recommendation for UV-Ray Treatment

If you want to achieve a lasting effect, you should go for ten to twelve illumination sessions. Light therapy cannot be replaced by the light found in standard solariums, which produce almost entirely UV-A rays.

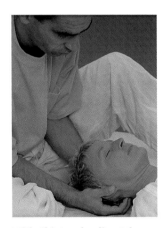

With Shiatsu, healing takes place through touch.

A Recommendation for Shiatsu Therapy

Shiatsu is especially appropriate for combating burnout, a hardening of the muscles, and blockages in the spine.

Shiatsu, the mobility of your body will improve, as will your posture.

Administration of the Therapy

Shiatsu massage therapists not only use their hands but also their underarms, knees, and feet, in order to create the desired pressure at certain points along the body. The treatment takes place on an exercise mat or on a large Japanese mat (about 10 by 13 feet, or 3 by 4 meters) on the floor. It requires quite a bit of sensitivity on the part of the therapist. A session usually lasts an hour.

Side Effects

If you have severe pains in your back, it might be difficult at first to work on the hard mat. However, this discomfort disappears after a few sessions, as your suppleness increases. Some people might feel uncomfortable with this type of intimate, intense physical work.

Areas of Application

❖ Hyperactivity, tension, inability to relax, nervousness
❖ Headaches and back pains
❖ Digestive problems and menstrual problems
❖ Muscular pain and tension
❖ Fatigue

Dr. Trager's Movement Therapy

Complete muscular relaxation

Milton Trager, M.D., from California, developed his movement therapy about forty years ago. It is a mild form of therapy that has as its goal the total relaxation of all the muscles. This therapy is a mental and physical learning process, consisting of two parts:
❖ The patient lies down passively. The therapist applies a number of rhythmic movement impulses in different directions that relate indirectly to all the muscles, including those with a deep layer of tension. In this form of therapy, the muscular release is not the result of a massage but of a learning process on the part of the nervous system.

❖ Certain physical exercises, which were developed by the mentalistic school of psychology (in contrast to that of behaviorism), are used in order to form a connection between particular visual images and complete physical relaxation. In this manner, over the course of time, the body learns to release muscle tension by means of visualization and imagination.

Administration of the Therapy

At a Trager therapy session, you lie down on a comfortably cushioned treatment table. It's best to wear light clothes. A physical therapist will gently rock you, loosen you up, and stretch you from head to toe with rhythmic movements. The session ends with exercises in which you are led through a number of simple movements as well as certain thoughts and images. A typical session takes from one to one and a half hours.

A Recommendation for Trager Movement Therapy
Going to a Trager session is like taking a short vacation. Treat yourself to this form of complete relaxation once or twice a month.

Side Effects

Some people have difficulty absorbing such mild movements. If you become dizzy—which is caused by the inner ear—then this therapy is not appropriate for you.

Areas of Application

❖ Aids in the healing process following a long period of bed rest
❖ Eases tension related to headaches, migraines, neck pains, back pains, pains that are related to posture, and sleep disturbances
❖ Helps in preventing osteoporosis

Also a preventive for osteoporosis

Manual Muscle Therapy (MM)

Manual muscle therapy is a complete treatment for problems related to the muscles, nerves, intervertebral disks, vertebrae, joints, and connective tissue, as well as diseases that derive from these types of problems. The basic concept behind manual muscle therapy is that the underlying cause of these diseases is long-term muscular tension. This tension is especially prevalent in the involuntary muscles.

A Recommendation for Manual Muscle Therapy

Many cases of disk damage are caused by tense muscles. In such cases, manual muscle therapy can prevent you from needing to have an operation. This method can also heal the pain that remains after an operation.

If a muscle is tense for an extended period of time, then the blood will not circulate enough in this muscle. Therefore, it cannot get enough oxygen, and this causes the tension to persist. In this way, a vicious cycle is created in the muscle, which can cause lifelong muscular tension.

A lasting tension of this type in the muscles of the spine and the joints (for example, in the pelvic muscles and the knees) can lead to bad posture, reduced athletic ability, blocked nerves, and extreme wear and tear on the vertebrae, intervertebral disks, and the surfaces of the joints. The bones are being pressed together so tightly it's as if they are being held in an iron fist. This is what causes certain disorders, such as slipped disks and arthritis, and their accompanying pain.

Administration of the Therapy

Tension in the spine, arms, and legs is treated with a vibrating motion administered by the hands. The positive effects of this treatment will disappear after a few hours to a few days if the muscles that relate to the tense muscles are not treated as well. The only way to get results with this form of therapy is to treat all the muscles that are related to the problem area. If some of the related muscles are not treated, then they will lead their tension back into the muscles that have been relaxed, causing the treated muscles to tense up again. A typical therapy session lasts up to one hour, and it is necessary to go to one to three sessions a week.

Warning

You should not undergo this therapy if you take a blood-thinning medication or if you are very sensitive to pain.

Side Effects

If you have a tendency to develop black-and-blue marks, nosebleeds, or bleeding in your gums, it would be advisable to take vitamin K before undergoing this form of treatment.

Areas of Application

❖ Damaged spine: intervertebral disk problems, spinning trauma, posture damage (scoliosis or kyphosis)

❖ Acute or chronic problems of the sciatic nerve
Arthritis in the hips or the knees, as well as pain follow-
ing operations on these joints
❖ Facial pains (trigeminal neuralgia)

Continuous Shower Therapy

Computer workstations, satellite televisions, and cellu-
lar phones are considered to be some of the most
advanced technical developments in our time. However,
along with them, there is an increase in the flow of rays,
which are loaded with energy and which go through
our bodies. Electromagnetic radiation loads the air with
electromagnetic particles (ions), especially those that are
positively charged. This radiation causes our bodies to
suffer from stress. We are overloaded both physically
and mentally, we feel tense, and our nerves are irritated.

We could balance the effects of this radiation by
going to places that are loaded with negative ions.
Examples of such places are mountains more than
4,920 feet (1,500 meters) in height, where the ultravio-
let rays of the sun create such an effect, or the vicinity
of the sea, where the swirling of the water releases negative ions. It is for this reason that we recover more
quickly when we are in the mountains or by the sea.

If you are looking for a place that will contain the
highest amount of negatively charged ions, you will find
it right beneath a waterfall. Continuous shower therapy
is an attempt to emulate this type of arrangement. The
body's release of an electric charge has proven to have a
clearly positive effect on the organism. All of the accu-
mulated poisons (toxins) in the tissue are led out of the
system, all the lymphatic blockages (edemas) are
released, and all muscular tension is completely
relieved. After a continuous shower, you will feel like
you have been reborn.

Administration of the Therapy

You lie down comfortably in the bathtub and receive a
fully automated massage from seven different shower
heads. The therapy lasts fifteen minutes on the back
and fifteen minutes on the stomach. The flow of warm
water is interrupted at times with thirty seconds of cold

A Recommendation for Continuous Shower Therapy

A continuous shower is
easy on the body, and it
is therefore appropriate
for even quite elderly
people. In cases of any
spinal problems or
lymphatic edemas, I
would recommend a
sequence of ten treat-
ments.

The imitation of a waterfall

water. This is done so that the circulation won't slow down too much. Of course, your head is turned away from the direct spray.

Side Effects

Continuous shower therapy can cause the blood pressure to lower slightly. For this reason, it is recommended that you lie down and relax for thirty to forty-five minutes after having the treatment. This form of therapy is not appropriate for people who suffer from claustrophobia.

Give yourself time to relax afterward.

Areas of Application

❖ Tension in the throat area, the chest, and the lumbar vertebrae
❖ Swelling after operations on the joints (such as knee or hip operations)
❖ All types of lymphatic blockages in the legs
❖ Release of stress and muscle tension
❖ Release of poisons through the skin, which is especially effective during fasting cures (detoxification of the blood through the skin)

Lymphatic Drainage

Lymphatic drainage is a massage of the skin that is performed on top of lymphatic tissue and veins. This gives support to the natural transporting processes of the body. It therefore helps to release edemas (lymphatic blockages), activates the autonomic nervous system, and can aid the body in developing immunity against local diseases.

A Recommendation for Lymphatic Drainage

Lymphatic drainage has far-reaching benefits. It has no side effects, and in many countries it is covered by health insurance.

Administration of the Therapy

The therapist massages either the entire body or just the chest and the stomach area in a circular motion. This serves to stimulate the lymph to flow in the direction of the heart. At the same time, blockages and waste products are released from the tissue. This form of therapy consists of twelve to eighteen sessions, which are administered at a rate of two or three a week.

Side Effects

If you suffer from cardiac insufficiency, it is recommended that you discuss this condition with your natural medicine practitioner. Otherwise, there are no known side effects.

Areas of Application

❖ All kinds of tension in the area of the spine
❖ All kinds of swelling and lymphatic blockage
❖ All sorts of pain, especially facial pain (trigeminal neuralgia), nerve-related pain, pain in the joints, and rheumatism in the softer parts of the body
❖ Removal of waste products as well as the stimulation of detoxification through the skin (especially during the course of a fasting cure)

Colon Hydrotherapy (Enema)

If the intestinal flora (see page 15) is damaged as a result of your eating something that did not agree with you or your taking medications, disease-causing bacteria and waste products will settle in. In such cases, an enema can be helpful. When the large intestine is cleansed of the rotten, fermented remains of the stools, it is detoxified and the immune system is relieved as a result. After the enema, you will feel refreshed, free, and relaxed, as well as a little tired.

A Recommendation for Colon Hydrotherapy

This is by far the best form of an enema. If you suffer from chronic constipation, it can be very helpful on a regular basis (once or twice a month).

Application of the Therapy

In colon hydrotherapy, the large intestine is flushed with filtered water at different temperatures. The temperature differences (between 82.4 and 98.6 degrees F, or 28 and 37 degrees C) are useful as a type of internal Kneipp therapy (see page 83) of the entire large intestine, which is being emptied out. Due to modern developments in the devices used in administering colon hydrotherapy, this form of therapy does not lead to any troubling or unpleasant odors.

Hygienic measures without any unpleasantness

The enema is followed by a sterile flushing action that leads in a one-way fashion into a closed system. The water that flows back out of the system—along with the rest of the stools—does so by a small window on the enema device on its way out, which allows the therapist to measure the amount, form, and nature of the contents of the intestine.

The administration of the therapy lasts from forty-five minutes to an hour. During the course of the therapy, it is not necessary to be in the vicinity of a bathroom. However, in the event that you feel the need to rid yourself of leftover fluids, it is recommended that you remain near a bathroom during the two hours following the therapy.

Side Effects

None. However, it should be noted that this method is not recommended after intestinal operations.

Areas of Application

❖ All sorts of intestinal problems that commonly accompany constipation
❖ Purification during the course of any type of fasting cure
❖ Useful in combating food and skin allergies

A Recommendation for Symbiotic Influence

If you have taken antibiotics three or more times over the course of a year, it would be a good idea to strengthen your intestinal flora by means of symbiotic influence.

Microbe Therapy (Symbiotic Influence)

With this therapy, a sample of the stools is sent to a laboratory, where the intestinal bacteria and fungi in the stools are cultivated in a special culture medium. This culture medium shows whether the bacteria and the fungi found in the intestines are a source of health or disease. A vaccine is created from the cultivation of the healthy bacteria to be used in each individual case. This vaccine supports the growth of the healthy intestinal flora and thus strengthens the overall immune system in the intestines.

Application of the Therapy

Adults take the vaccine on a weekly basis in the form of an injection under the skin. Children receive this therapy in the form of drops.

Side Effects

It is possible that you will experience a strong reddening of the skin. However, you can prevent this side effect by having the vaccine thinned out.

Areas of Application

❖ Tendency to develop infections
❖ Chronic immune deficiency
❖ Settlement of intestinal fungi
❖ As a supplemental treatment in combating allergies

Vitamin-B Therapy

Vitamins from the B-complex group improve the energetic metabolism, especially that of the liver. This is of special importance in cases of fatigue (see pages 20 and 45). Vitamins B-6 and B-12 and folic acid improve regeneration. Vitamin B-6 is important for protein metabolism as well as for the functioning of the nervous system. Vitamin B-12 plays a key role in the creation of red blood corpuscles, which are responsible for the transportation of oxygen in the blood.

A Recommendation for Vitamin-B Therapy

This form of therapy works rapidly and is highly effective. It is especially recommended in cases of physical and mental exhaustion from overworking, for recovery from diseases and operations, and for children and adolescents—as well as adults—who have difficulties learning and concentrating.

Application of the Therapy

A treatment cycle consists of twelve injections, which are administered in the muscle (preferably in the buttock) and are given two or three times a week. The injections supply the body with enough substance for an entire year. Therefore, after one year, the treatment should be repeated. This therapy is a must for patients who have had stomach-reduction operations, because they cause a chronic vitamin-B deficiency.

Side Effects

As with every medication, certain allergies and skin irritations might develop. Injections into the veins could cause light headaches.

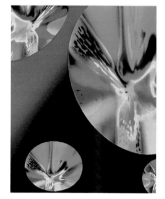

The beauty of the vitamin-B crystal can be seen under a microscope.

Areas of Application

❖ Fatigue
❖ Anemia
❖ Pains in the nerves and infections of the nerves
❖ Liver diseases, alcohol problems
❖ Stomach and intestinal problems
❖ After taking antibiotics

Thymus Therapy

The thymus gland in human beings is located behind the breastbone, and it is an important part of the immune system (see drawing on page 22). When we are about thirty years of age, the thymus gland decreases its activity, depending on the stress level of the individual. In severe cases, this is manifested as an immune system deficiency. When this occurs, it is helpful to support the immune system with animal thymus remedies. These are usually made up from excretions of the thymus gland in young calves and are used as a substitute for the inactive components of the human gland. In contrast to fresh cell therapy, in this case the organ extracts are not administered directly into the human body but are tested on a carrier (such as BSE) in a laboratory, after which they are stored in ampules or as pills.

A Recommendation for Thymus Therapy

Every elderly person who suffers from a deficiency in his or her immune system would benefit greatly from this form of therapy.

Application of the Therapy

You should take two pills two or three times a day. If the therapy is being administered in the form of injections, then you should take two ampules two or three times a week as an injection in the buttock. The entire therapy should consist of twenty ampules.

Side Effects

If your thyroid gland does not function at a sufficient level, if your thymus gland shows evidence of hyperfunctioning, or if you have an allergy to beef protein, then you should not undergo this form of therapy. It is also not advised for people who are on long-term cortisone treatment or for pregnant women or new mothers who are breast-feeding.

Areas of Application

❖ Stimulation of the immune system in cases of immune deficiency
❖ Strengthening of your general immunity and your ability to recuperate
❖ Helpful against infectious rheumatic diseases
❖ Beneficial as a supplemental therapy in the treatment of cancer, as well as for the damage caused by radioactive treatment, chemotherapy, or cortisone therapy

Homeopathy

Homeopathy was developed by Samuel Hahnemann in 1785. In this form of therapy, every person and his or her symptoms are taken into consideration on an individual basis. There are no remedies for specific illnesses, such as the flu. Two people who suffer from the same type of flu will usually receive two different remedies, because their complaints probably will not be exactly the same. Homeopathy attributes a special importance to the symptoms. If you are interested in pursuing a cure with homeopathy, I suggest that you read up on it further—there are many books specifically on the subject.

A Recommendation for Homeopathy

Outside of a case in which an organ cannot be saved, homeopathy would be the preferred treatment for most diseases because it has the least amount of side effects.

Administration of the Therapy

In a conversation with a homeopathic practitioner about the history of your illness (a case history), you will be asked about all the details concerning the symptoms of your illness, such as: Do you suffer from fevers with or without sweating? At what time of day do you feel worse? Have you become sensitive to light or to anything else? The conversation can take anywhere from ten minutes to two hours.
❖ Classical homeopathy looks for the one remedy that will take care of all the symptoms at once. This remedy may come in the form of milk-sugar capsules.
❖ Nonclassical homeopathy uses a combination of various remedies at once.

An initial conversation with a homeopathic practitioner can last up to two hours.

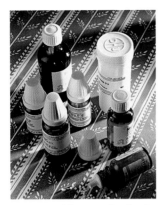

Homeopathic remedies in the form of tinctures, tablets, and milk-sugar capsules

There is a very successful line of new homeopathic remedies from Spain for the treatment of fatigue, and they come in the form of ampules. These remedies stimulate specific organs and have an influence on the metabolism of protein.

Side Effects

For a short period of time, the symptoms might worsen, but this is considered to be proof that the appropriate remedy has been chosen.

Areas of Application

❖ All functional and autonomic disturbances
❖ Enhancement of your immunity in cases of immune deficiency
❖ Flu-related infections
❖ Chronic infections
❖ Hormonal imbalance

Acupuncture

A Recommendation for Acupuncture

Migraines and pains of this sort can be treated very effectively by acupuncture.

Acupuncture is a form of diagnosis and therapy that was developed in China more than 2,000 years ago. It is based on thousands of years of observing the correlation among various parts of the human body. The organ clock (see drawing on page 47) is a result of these observations.

Acupuncture is based on the assumption that there is a stream of energy that flows through the twelve organs of the body within two hours. The meridians are the tracks through which this energy flows. Diseases are seen as blockages along this stream of energy.

The organ clock shows the time of day at which the various organs experience maximal energy flow. Health problems that repeatedly appear at a certain time of the day indicate a specific organ—for example, sleep disturbances between 1 and 3 in the morning point to the liver (see organ clock on page 47).

For a deeper understanding of this form of alternative medicine, I suggest that you seek further information in the many books specifically on the subject. Acupuncture has proven to be so effective that a number of health insurance companies now cover the costs of this treatment.

Application of the Therapy

Very fine needles (in acupuncture) or finger pressure (in acupressure) is applied to certain points on the skin, in order to release blockages of the energy flow and return the body to a healthy balance.

Side Effects

If the therapist makes a mistake and leads the energy in the wrong direction, you might experience a worsening of the symptoms.

Areas of Application

❖ All kinds of pain (especially migraines, back pain, intestinal cramps)
❖ Fatigue
❖ Asthma
❖ Inability to tolerate medications

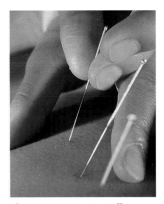

The acupuncture needles are so thin that their insertion rarely stings or causes bleeding.

Mora, or Bio-resonance, Therapy

This modern natural therapy is based on the philosophy of acupuncture (see opposite page). However, the energy streams are altered on the basis of their frequencies.

Application of the Therapy

The negative frequencies of a sick organ are measured and neutralized or exchanged with positive frequencies. These frequencies are applied in the form of weak electricity through electrodes that are placed on the skin.

Side Effects

There are no known side effects.

Areas of Application

❖ All kinds of allergies (especially allergic asthma, hay fever, allergic dermatitis)
❖ Regulation of the metabolic system
❖ Acceleration of healing processes

A Recommendation for Mora Therapy

Mora therapy has proven its effectiveness with allergies that cannot be cured in any other way.

The Cost of Naturopathic Treatment

There are no preset prices for natural medicine treatments. The cost varies according to the quality, the time required, the regional price levels, and the competition. The following price list displays the average costs, so that you will have a general idea regarding the price range.

How Much Does Your Insurance Cover?

The current cost cuts at many health insurance companies make it difficult to estimate which treatments will be covered by health insurance in the near future. Generally, insurance companies cover conventional medicine (physician care, hospitalization, and medication) but are less prone to pay for alternative forms of treatment. Many health insurance companies try to rid themselves of their responsibility to pay for naturopathic

The Prices of Naturopathic Therapies

Therapy	Price
Decoder demography (DD)	$46 to $76 (30 min.)
Thermoregulation diagnosis (TRD)	$50 to $105 (30 min.)
Bio-dynamic protein profile	$115 to $150 (blood work)
Bioelectronics of Vincent (BEV)	$40 to $78 (blood, mucous, and urine tests)
Candida immune profile	$80 to $115 (blood work)
Blood ozone therapy (infusions)	$50 to $85 (20 to 30 min.)
Oxygen inhalation of Prof. Ardenne (ionized)	$15 to $28 (15 min.)
Illumination with UV light	$40 to $105 (20 to 45 min.)
Shiatsu therapy	$85 to $95 (one hour)
Trager movement therapy	$85 to $105 (1 to 1.5 hours)
Manual muscle therapy	$85 to $100 (1 hour)
Continuous shower therapy	$30 to $65 (30 min.)
Lymphatic drainage	$25 to $48 (20 to 45 min.)
Colon hydrotherapy	$50 to $95 (30 to 60 min.)
Vitamin-B therapy	$8 to $15 (injection)
Thymus therapy	$15 to $60 (injection of varied potency)
Acupuncture	$25 to $90 (depending on the amount of time)
Homeopathy	$40 to $205 (depending on the amount of time)

treatment, with the excuse that there is not enough evidence to prove the effectiveness of alternative medicine. When there is no clear proof concerning the efficacy of a certain therapy, the assumption is that this therapy is not effective and thus there is no medical necessity for the treatment.

If you are too disabled to work and have to take out a private health insurance policy, you need to be aware that most insurance companies exclude payment for "preexisting conditions." Therefore, if you have already accrued a slew of medical bills for the diagnosis and treatment of chronic fatigue syndrome, it will be difficult to find an affordable insurance policy, to say nothing of one that covers natural medicine.

Many people with CFS are too ill to work, so they lose their health benefits.

Some people who have private insurance plans have chosen the following solution: They select an insurance program in which the deductible is very high (around $5,000 a year) so that the insurance only pays whatever amount exceeds the deductible. This way, the monthly payments are more manageable. With the money that they end up saving every month, they can finance their natural therapies and avoid the nerve-wracking ordeal of having to negotiate with their insurance companies.

A tip for people with private insurance

It's also important to know that in the United States if you have medically documented chronic fatigue syndrome, you are probably entitled to Social Security disability benefits. In fact, a recent ruling issued by the Social Security Administration should make it easier for disabled people with CFS to acquire benefits at an earlier stage in the appeals process.

What You Can Do Yourself

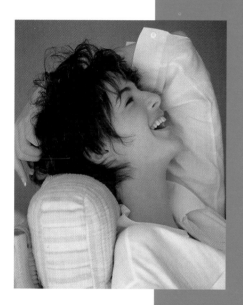

Self-initiation is the most important component in maintaining your health. In the following chapter, I would like to show you how diverse and pleasurable this component can be when you allow yourself time to enjoy your desires, your fantasies, and your creativity, and when you begin with the phrase "I want . . ."

You Are in Command

Your approach to your health is totally in your own hands. No one can take this responsibility away from you. But how can you turn what may seem like an obligation into a choice? This is what I would like to explore in the present chapter. Let yourself be inspired by what you read, and engage your creativity to invent your own water treatments, energy drinks, images for meditation, and different kinds of physical exercise.

How to Relieve Yourself of Stress

You can acquire a few simple mental skills that will help you get your stress under control. This can be very helpful when you are dealing with burnout.

Motivation in Reaching Your Goal

In order to reach your goal of decreasing your level of stress, it is not enough to wish for the stress to go away—this must be a longing of your entire being. Therefore, it is important to be clear with yourself by answering these questions: Is finally being rid of the destructive stress in your life truly your goal? Is this goal realistic and attainable? Can you set a date by which you want to reach this goal? If your answers to these questions are yes, then you can realistically start to believe in the possibility of your success. You will need to write up an agreement with yourself (see page 78), which should include the date and your signature. Set precise and systematic targets for yourself, and rate your progress in relation to them. In order to do this, you will need to answer the following questions:

❖ Where do you experience the most stress? (On your way to work? While you are shopping? During your free time? While keeping to a tight schedule? When taking too much work upon yourself? While performing household chores? While educating your children? During the course of organizing your daily schedule? In connection with financial difficulties? Or in the context of an intimate relationship?)

❖ What is the cause of the stress? (Is it that you can't say no because you want to think highly of yourself or you want to get validation from others? Think about why you take so much upon yourself.)

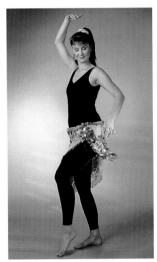

Belly dancing: A creative form of movement that feels good physically and thus promotes recovery

Ask yourself these questions.

An Agreement with Myself (for a Period of at Least One Week)

I promise myself to try to prevent any situations of stress from occurring in my life for at least seven days, and to write down and analyze the kinds of stress that do affect me during this period, regardless of the emotions that come up as a result of the success or the failure of my efforts.

I am prepared to receive criticism and less attention from the people around me.

I know that it is not realistic to expect myself to experience success in attaining inner calm and a new orientation in my life before the end of this week.

If I give up before the end of this week, I am aware of the fact that I am not granting myself a fair chance in successfully combating my stress.

I agree to try to reduce the stress factors in my life and to write down an analysis of stresses when they come up until ———————— (exact date).

——————————————————— Date, Signature

Change this proposed text in accordance with your own needs.

❖ What self-image have I created for myself? (Which one of the personality types in the anagram (see page 37) do I fit into? Which one do I want to become? How can I escape the addiction of needing approval?)

❖ Which changes in my life am I capable of making on a short-term basis? Which ones can I make on a long-term basis? (Write down your answers, so that in one year you will be able to monitor your long-term progress.)

The Raisins Exercise

Before you read through this exercise, you'll need to get three raisins. You can also use nuts that are cracked and ready to be eaten. Are you ready? Then let's begin:

First get out three raisins.

❖ Observe each raisin as if you had never seen raisins before in your life: Pay attention to the color, the skin, the composition, and other traits.

❖ What thoughts and images come up in your mind with regard to the raisins? Are they pleasant or unpleasant?

❖ Allow yourself time in order to become aware of the actual smell of the raisins. Pay attention to the increasing saliva in your mouth.

❖ Focus your attention on your arm as it gradually moves your hand holding one of the raisins toward your mouth. Concentrate on the fingers that slowly place the raisin in your mouth.

Allow yourself plenty of time.

❖ Chew on the raisin very slowly. Experience the taste very intensely.

❖ As soon as you recognize the wish to swallow the raisin, register this impulse in your conscious mind; experience it from the moment it pops up in your thoughts until the moment at which the raisin disappears in your stomach.

❖ Observe yourself carefully. Imagine that the only change that has occurred in your body is that it now contains this raisin.

❖ Eat the other two raisins in the same conscious manner.

Results of Conscious Eating

You have just completed the "conscious eating" exercise, in which you consciously experienced the taste of a raisin, perhaps for the first time in your life. You may have caught yourself wanting to reach for the next raisin before you had finished eating the one in your mouth. Did it become clear to you how little attention you usually pay to the food that you eat? Nevertheless, you succeeded in:

The present moment, the here and now, is the only moment there is.

❖ Shutting out any external stress factors
❖ Not thinking of anything else
❖ Only doing one thing at a time
❖ Relieving yourself of stress while doing the exercise

Meditation: A Means of Combating Stress

Stress always starts with thinking (see page 13). Getting rid of stress must therefore begin with a mental process of switching off. Meditation is an excellent method for doing this, and it can easily be incorporated into your daily life.

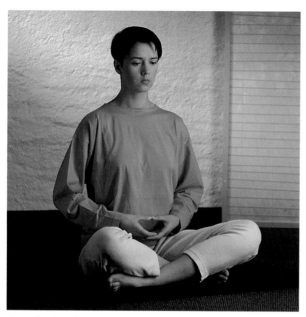

In order to relax, concentrate on your breathing.

This Is How You Do It

First, it's important to create a relaxing atmosphere. If necessary, turn off the ringer of your phone and disconnect the doorbell; you might also want to close the windows and put on some quiet meditative music to block out the noises from the street. Sit on a chair, a meditation pillow, or a meditation bench, or simply sit on the floor. Sit upright with a straight spine, in order to prevent any back pain. Lay your hands softly in your lap, with the palms facing upward.

Read each of the sentences below aloud. Read them in their complete form, and repeat them at least three times. Then close your eyes (or keep them open slightly) and think about the short form of the sentences with every breath that you take. Concentrate on your breath and on the image of the short form of the sentence. It will take only a few minutes for you to feel the inner calm and relaxation that can be obtained by doing this meditation exercise.

Exercise Sentences for Zen Meditation

Long Form	Short Form
While breathing in—I am aware of breathing in	In
While breathing out—I am aware of breathing out	Out
Breathing in—I see myself as a flower	Flower
Breathing out—I feel fresh	Fresh
Breathing in—I see myself as a mountain	Mountain
Breathing out—I feel solid	Solid
Breathing in—I see myself as calm water	Water
Breathing out—I reflect the things around me as they are	Reflection
Breathing in—I see myself as open space	Space
Breathing out—I feel free	Free

Telephone Meditation

This is another form of meditation that is very effective in combating stress in daily life. Every time the phone rings, take a minute to breathe in and out three times, thinking of the following:

Meditation is an exercise of the mind for the purpose of obtaining peace, happiness, and harmony for oneself and for other people.

Sentences for Telephone Meditation

Long Form	Short Form
Breathing in—I experience peace	Peace
Breathing out—I smile to myself	Smile

Something else that you can do is hang a mirror above your telephone with a sign that says "Please smile." This way, you will be able to check yourself, and it will be a reminder to do the phone meditation at the same time. Try performing this exercise every time the phone rings. You will be rewarded for this small effort by being more relaxed on the phone and having more satisfying conversations. The people on the other end of the line will feel your smile, recognize your inner balance, and probably be more relaxed themselves, saying things that otherwise they might have forgotten due to the hectic pace of their daily lives.

The Importance of Physical Exercise

A lack of physical exercise combined with physical and emotional stress is bound to lead to bad posture and painful muscular tension. The resulting limitations in physical mobility often bring on mental laziness. Physical exercise can help you in restoring the balance between body and soul. However, in comparing sports that are geared toward increasing stamina and competitive sports, it is clear that the first type can strengthen the immune system whereas the latter type can weaken it. What factors make the difference?

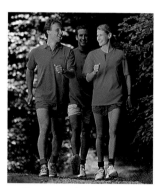

Walking: A form of aerobic exercise that strengthens the immune system

Aerobic and Anaerobic Exercise

"Aerobic" refers to anything that has to do with the presence of air (oxygen), whereas "anaerobic" concerns any-

Important: Sustain your activity for more than fifteen minutes.

thing that takes place without air. When large groups of muscles are set in motion for an extended period of time (fifteen minutes or longer), this causes you to breathe more deeply, increases your heart rate, and provides a better oxygen supply to the muscles. This kind of exercise is called "aerobic" exercise. Aerobic exercise strengthens the immune system. On the other hand, when it comes to a high level of performance in competitive sports, the muscles use more oxygen than the blood, heart, and lungs are able to produce. The outcome is an inadequate provision of oxygen to the muscles, which is an anaerobic state. This causes a weakening of the immune system. As a result, professional athletes often suffer from an immune deficiency combined with an increased frequency of infections.

Weight Loss through Aerobic Exercise

It is very interesting to observe the results of measuring a person's energy level after performing aerobic exercises. Thirty minutes of aerobic exercise are followed by up to fifteen hours of energy consumption in the body. The reason for this is that the exercise causes an increase in inner activity, which in turn burns fat for an extended period of time.

I have observed in my clinic that aerobic exercises that last sixty minutes will make people lose one pound, whereas when they perform ninety minutes of aerobic exercise it is possible for them to take off more than 2 pounds. On the other hand, the first fifteen minutes of aerobic exercise do not lead to any loss of weight at all! During the first fifteen minutes, only the fat reserves of the liver are being used, not the excess fat on the hips and the legs. Therefore, if you wish to lose weight, it doesn't make sense to jog four times a day for fifteen minutes.

Warning for People with Heart Disease

If you suffer from angina pectoris, you should consult your doctor before setting out on an athletic regime.

Appropriate Exercises

Whether for the purpose of relaxing, increasing the strength of your immune system, or losing weight, appropriate aerobic exercises include any kind of sport that enhances your stamina, such as fast walking, running, cycling, rowing, or skiing. Don't take too many breaks, and be sure not to turn it into a competitive sport! You are on the right track if your pulse (beats per minute) remains at the ideal level for your age group for a period of thirty to forty-five minutes. It is recommended that you perform those exercises that increase your stamina two to three times a week. Measure your pulse every ten minutes.

It would be ideal to measure your pulse with a mechanism designed specifically for this purpose. There are simple devices that can be connected to the ear with clips. Better devices come with a belt that contains a transmitter and a receiver. They keep a record of the amount of time that you were in the target area as well as exceeded the target area. In this way, you can document your achievements.

Target Level and Ideal Pulse Level during Aerobic Exercise

Age	Target Level (pulse beats per minute)	Ideal Level (pulse beats per minute)
20	130–170	140
25	127–166	137
30	124–162	133
35	120–157	130
40	117–153	127
45	114–149	123
50	111–145	119
55	107–140	116
60	104–136	112
65	101–132	109
70	95–128	105

Start the Day Feeling Fresh—with Water

Water is one of the four basic elements. There is no life without water. Water symbolizes both an untamed power as well as a yielding softness. Water heals the body (see page 65) and caresses the soul; therefore, we go to places that have water—such as steam baths, swimming pools, saunas, and thermal baths—in order to relax, recuperate, and mentally recharge ourselves. Take advantage of all these possibilities in the area where you live, and go on trips to more distant water attractions as well. Moreover, try the measures, which will be introduced in the follwing sections, that are performed right in your own home.

Measuring Your Pulse

Count your pulse on the inner side of your wrist for fifteen seconds; then multiply it by four. This is how you can obtain the measurement of your pulse per minute.

Kneipp Water Treatments

About a century ago, a priest by the name of Sebastian Kneipp developed an exciting and very successful form of therapy that uses water in a variety of ways. Kneipp water treatments go far beyond practices that are held to be common knowledge. They are an all-encompassing form of therapy that is based on the following five pillars: water, order, movement, nutrition, and healing herbs. When you perform any of these treatments, please pay attention to the basic rules for using water (see highlighted text in box).

Cool Arm Bath

Start your day by bathing your hands in cool water in the sink:

❖ Fill up the sink with cool water (approximately 64.4 degrees F, or 18 degrees C).

❖ Place your warm hands and underarms in the water several times for a couple of minutes each time. You will feel an immediate reaction in your legs. This means that by bathing your arms you have achieved an increase in the circulation in your legs as well.

Knee Spray

It's best to stand in the bathtub for this form of water therapy, and you will need the assistance of a friend. If this is not possible, you can also carry out this procedure yourself while seated on the rim of the tub. The following parts of the body are sprayed with water from the hand nozzle in the manner indicated:

❖ From the back of the right foot to the right knee and back again

❖ From the back of the left foot to the left knee and back again

❖ From behind the heel of the right foot to the hollow of the right knee and back again

❖ From behind the heel of the left foot to the hollow of the left knee and back again

In the morning, perform the knee spray with water that is somewhere between warm (86 degrees F, or 30 degrees C) and hot (98.6 to 104 degrees F, or 37 to 40 degrees C); in the evening, the water should be somewhere between cool (68 degrees F, or 20 degrees C) and cold (59 degrees F, or 15 degrees C). After a week,

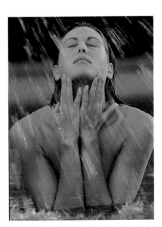

Water therapy heals the body and caresses the soul.

Basic Rules for Using Water

❖ Begin the treatment with an area of the body that is far from the area that is sick. The sick area will automatically react along with this secondary area.

❖ Do not use cold water on areas of the body that are cold. If it is necessary to use cold water, make sure that you warm up these areas beforehand.

❖ Start with small splashes, and build them up gradually, just as you would do with any training that is to be built up slowly.

❖ If you are sensitive to temperature changes, start with warm water and then gradually move to cold water by alternating with warm water.

reverse the rhythm of the therapy. In the morning, change from hot to cold (two minutes hot, thirty seconds cold), and, in the evening, use either warm or hot water.

The Kneipp Fresh Shower

When you get up in the morning, take a warm shower for a couple of minutes until you feel good and warm all over.

Warning

If you have an infection of any sort, you should not perform Kneipp water therapy. Do not bathe in cold water during menstruation or if you have a urinary tract infection (such as a bladder infection or prostate problems). If you have any hesitations, ask your doctor whether or not you should use the water-healing method and, if so, when.

Then lead the hand nozzle—spraying cold water—from the back side of your right foot, over the knee, the hip, the stomach, and the chest, up to the throat. Repeat the same order on the left side of your body. Next, lead the water stream from the right heel all the way to the right shoulder, and then from the left heel to the left shoulder. At the end, spray a strong stream of cold water over both shoulders from both the front and the back. Then dry yourself off with a towel.

Other Possible Uses of Water

Let yourself be inspired to do the following:
❖ Run barefoot over a meadow that is covered with dew
❖ Use brushes while bathing
❖ Take whirlpool baths, mustard footbaths, and bubble baths with herbal extracts (followed by thirty minutes of relaxation)
❖ Rub your body with dry snow in winter

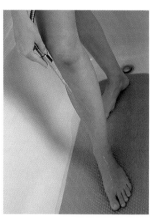

The knee spray is a favorite, because it is so simple to perform.

Sauna

The sauna, which was developed in Finland, is not part of Kneipp therapy, although it has similar effects: It toughens you up, purifies you, detoxifies you, and helps to release stress. When you sit in a sauna, the temperature inside your body increases by a couple of degrees, as it does when you have a slight fever. This leads to an increase in the mucous secretions in the breathing passages, which cleans out the breathing apparatus. Regular visits to the sauna (once a week, for two to three cycles, the first ones without infusion) stimulate the immune system and protect the body against colds.

Warning

If you are sick with the flu, angina, a sinus infection, or bronchitis, do not go to the sauna for a period of eight to ten days. If you do not avoid the sauna during this time, the overheating of the lungs can cause pneumonia.

Drinks That Make You Fit: Energy Cocktails

I would like to acquaint you with a few energy cocktails (and dishes) that can serve as a quick pickup for days when you feel exhausted or down. The vitamins in these cocktails are very helpful in counteracting any kind of energy loss, immune deficiency, or result of stress.

Exotic Fruit Salad (for two people)

½ honeydew melon
1 slice pineapple
1 kiwi
Juice from ½ lemon
1 tablespoon shelled pistachios
1 tablespoon pine nuts
Fresh ginger

Cut the fruit into small pieces, add the lemon juice, and then season the mixture with the fresh ginger. Cover the mixture, letting it absorb the flavors. Place the fruit in two large wineglasses. Then decorate with the pine nuts and the finely chopped pistachios.

Melon Yogurt (for two people)

½ honeydew melon
Juice from ½ lemon
1 cup plain yogurt
2 mint leaves for decoration

Remove the seeds from the honeydew melon, take the fruit out of the rind, and mix it in a blender, together with the lemon juice and the yogurt. If necessary, you can add sugar. Decorate each portion with a mint leaf. Tip: You can turn this dish into a refreshing summer drink by adding spring water and crushed ice.

Mango Drink (for two people)

1 fresh mango
¼ quart (or liter) orange juice
Juice from 1 lemon
Sparkling spring water

Peel the mango, reserving two pieces with the peel for decoration. Remove the pit, and puree the fruit in a blender. Add the lemon juice and the orange juice with some sugar or other sweetener and some sparkling spring water.

Currant Mixture (for when you are in a hurry)

1 bottle currant juice
1 bottle bitter lemon

Mix equal amounts of currant juice and bitter lemon, and serve cold. This is a fruity drink rich in vitamin C.

Four-Fruits Juice (for four people)

Extracted juice from ½ pound apples, or ½ quart (liter) of apple juice

Puree the freshly washed strawberries in a blender; add the orange juice and the lemon juice as well as the juice that was extracted from the apples (or the apple juice).

Flavor the mixture with the vanilla sugar and the almond oil, and mix it all together. Decorate the drinks with a mint leaf, and, if you so desire, serve them with ice cream.

1 pound strawberries
Juice from 1 lemon
Juice from 2 oranges
2 tablespoons vanilla sugar
A few drops almond oil
4 mint leaves for decoration

Asian Cool (for two people)

Peel the fruit, and puree in a blender. Add the lemon juice and the honey, and then the water. The best choice would be a 0.75 quart (liter) bottle of carbonated spring water. Adding a few drops of angostura will give the drink a special, slightly bitter taste.

1 mango
1 pineapple
1 papaya
1 tablespoon lemon juice
1 tablespoon honey
1 bottle spring water

Kiwi Star (for two people)

Puree the peeled kiwis in a blender, and pass the mixture through a sieve. Pour into two glasses, and then pour the bitter lemon on top.

3 kiwis
¼ quart (liter) bitter lemon

Grapefruit Drink (for two people)

Mix the juices and some crushed ice in a blender. Divide the mixture into two glasses, and then pour the bitter lemon over each one.

¾ cup grapefruit juice
½ cup pineapple juice
A little over 2 tablespoons grenadine
¾ cup bitter lemon

Herbal Therapy (Phytotherapy)

We have a tradition of treatment achieved with herbal teas and compresses that goes back thousands of years. Today, most of these herbs can be obtained in the form of tablets or capsules. With them, the dosages are much more exact and the effectiveness is more reliable. If you follow the recommended dosages, you can take these remedies without any worries. However, if you wish to combine various remedies, it would be a good idea to consult a therapist.

Pheasant's-Eye, Lily of the Valley, Oleander, Squill

A purely herbal stimulation of the circulatory system—which is especially effective in cases of low blood pressure—is created through a combination of these four herbs. This blend is particularly helpful if you experience dizziness after standing up or if you have a cold.

Recommended dosage: Take one tablet two or three times a day for a period of six months, or according to your personal needs.

Artichoke

Recommended dosage: Take two 500 mg tablets twice a day at lunch and dinner. The duration of the treatment is determined by your personal needs.

Whoever doesn't care for the French artichoke schnapps Cynar can get the same artichoke concentration without the alcohol in the form of gallbladder pills. They help in combating digestive problems, flatulence, and fatigue, especially after eating. They are also useful if your cholesterol level is low.

Valerian (Catnip)

Recommended dosage: One 50 mg capsule two or three times a day will calm you down. For sleep, you should take three or four tablets one hour before bedtime. The duration of the therapy is determined by your personal needs.

Valerian can be found growing at the moist edges of forests and alongside running water. The root is effective in counteracting internal unrest, agitation, bad moods, problems falling asleep due to nervousness, and difficulties sleeping through the night. Not only does valerian have a relaxing effect and make you feel good, but it also balances out the autonomic nervous system.

Ginseng

Recommended dosage: Take four 50 mg capsules in the morning and at noon on a daily basis for a period of six months.

The ginseng root has been used for ages for a number of purposes, including strengthening oneself in cases of general tiredness and weakness, counteracting a reduced performance level or ability to concentrate, and aiding one's recovery from an illness (the convalescence stage). The daily dosage is between 400 mg and 1,800 mg. Unfortunately, there are a lot of products on the market that contain hardly any ginseng at all. For this reason, when shopping for ginseng pay attention to the amount of the active ingredient that the products contain.

Ginkgo Biloba

Recommended dosage: Take one 100 mg capsule twice a day or one 80 mg capsule two or three times a day. This herb can be consumed over a duration of several years.

This substance is excreted by the leaves of the ginkgo tree. It improves the circulation and, as a result, the nourishment of the tissue. Therefore, ginkgo products are used to combat a reduced performance level (both physical and intellectual), to increase your alertness and ability to wake up, and to strengthen your memory. Inexpensive products that contain 40 mg or less do not show any visible effects.

Saint-John's-Wort

Recommended dosage: Take one or two 200 mg capsules three times a day over a period of at least three to four months.

This is the best product for the purpose of combating the fatigue caused by depression (especially during menopause). However, in such cases, it takes three weeks for the optimal effects to take place. The effect is faster in cases of fear and nervous conditions, such as stomachaches caused by anxiety.

Kava Kava

Extracts from the root of this peppery plant, which makes its home around the South Seas, help primarily in situations of nervous fear, tension, and restlessness. It has no effect of drowsiness, so your performance level can be maintained at its fullest. This makes kava kava appropriate for use in combating fear before exams, stage fright, and all other types of stress related to nervous anticipation.

Recommended dosage: Take one 100 mg capsule two or three times a day over a period of two to three months.

Garlic

The active component in garlic can help improve a lack of motivation or concentration difficulties—particularly in older people—caused by circulatory disorders. It is also very helpful in alleviating metabolic problems. Garlic binds poisonous heavy metals, such as lead and cadmium, and it is effective against bacteria as well as free radicals (see page 23).

Recommended dosage: Take one or two finely chopped garlic cloves a day or one 280 mg capsule two to three times a day. Garlic can be taken over a period of several years.

Milk Thistle

This member of the aster family is an unbeatable remedy for treating liver problems (see page 20). It strengthens the liver, the gallbladder, and the entire digestive system. However, this herb can lose its effectiveness if less than the recommended dosage is taken. It is suggested to use this therapy for an extended duration, because the metabolism of the liver takes a long time to change.

Recommended dosage: Take one 165 mg capsule twice a day over a period of one to two years.

Nutmeg Flower

In ancient Egypt, this herb was already known as a revitalizing remedy. Nutmeg-flower capsules can be taken to harmonize the immune system and are ideal for cases of autonomic fatigue (see page 13), stomach and intestinal problems, and difficulties in sleeping through the night. They also help in the treatment of skin disorders (such as acne, psoriasis, and skin fungus), diseases of the breathing apparatus (such as bronchitis) and the joints, infections, and allergies (including hay fever, dermatitis, and allergic asthma).

Recommended dosage: Take one 450 mg capsule three times a day. For allergies, take two capsules two or three times a day over a duration of at least six months.

Recommended dosage: Take two 20 mg tablets twice a day over a period of at least one year.

Black Cohosh (Genus Cimicifuga)

Products that are made from this herb are appropriate for women suffering during menopause from hot flashes, excessive sweating, and depression, or from psycho-autonomic problems, such as being burnt out, feeling inner tension, being irritated, having difficulties concentrating, insomnia, and general fears and nervous restlessness.

Hawthorn

Recommended dosage: Take one 450 mg tablet once or twice a day. Hawthorn can be consumed over a duration of several years.

Hawthorn improves the blood circulation of the heart's coronary vessels so that the heart muscle receives more blood and oxygen. This is why hawthorn can be helpful in the following cases: fatigue caused by circulatory problems, a decrease in performance ability, circulatory disorders, and circulatory problems of the heart after infections or during periods of recovery from illnesses.

A nutritional consultation is recommended when:

❖ You are constantly exhausted or tired
❖ Your performance level has decreased although you are in the prime of your life
❖ Physical and emotional problems appear
❖ You are overweight or underweight
❖ Your general state of mind is that of wishing for improvement

Nutritional Supplements

I have already discussed the various kinds of nutritional deficiencies and the importance of a balanced diet (see pages 22 and 47). The appropriate diet for you, however, depends on your individual situation (past diseases, lifestyle, how much exercise you get, and so forth). For this reason, it is better to have a personal consultation with a nutritionist than to allow yourself to be guided by general ideas, and there are many nutritionists who offer this service.

Nevertheless, I don't want to miss this opportunity to acquaint you with some of the lesser-known nutritional supplements that are especially helpful in overcoming fatigue. They are usually effective due to their ability to stimulate the circulation, the metabolism, and the immune system. With the assistance of these supplements, it is possible to prevent a sudden crisis and achieve a lasting improvement. However, it's important to understand that these supplements when used alone are not sufficient in counteracting chronic burnout—they are helpful only in conjunction with other forms of therapy.

The following suggested remedies can be obtained at health food stores and drugstores or through mail-order catalogs, which are usually less expensive. You can take them without hesitation, as long as you follow the recommendations regarding dosage and length of treatment.

Adenosine

Adenosine triphosphate (ATP) is the biological keeper of energy. It allows restored energy to be released within seconds. This is especially true of energy that is stored in the muscles. Adenosine, which is one of the building blocks of ATP, is an energizer for anyone who suffers from stress-related fatigue. Adenosine improves the circulation and increases the supply of oxygen to the cells (see page 81).

Recommended dosage: Take one or two 20 mg capsules in the morning over a period of two to three months.

Bromelain and Papain

Bromelain and papain are proteins (enzymes) that are involved with many important processes in metabolism and the immune system. This is the reason that they can also be used medically for:

❖ A number of different infections accompanied by swelling (edemas, colds, sinus infections, bronchitis) Infections in the stomach area

❖ Infections in the veins, pains in the legs that result from a circulatory deficiency, lymphatic swelling, and skin infections

❖ Rheumatism in the softer parts of the body, and infectious phases of degenerative joint diseases and spine diseases

❖ Athletic injuries and bruises, recovery after operations, and recovery after tooth extractions

An abundance of bromelain and papain can be found in pineapples and papayas. However, because you cannot eat a whole pineapple every day, you should take the appropriate preparation.

Recommended dosage: Take ten tablets with 20 mg bromelain and 10 mg papain two or three times a day. In acute cases of bronchitis or sinus infection, take four tablets three or four times a day over a period of one week, followed by two tablets three times a day for two weeks.

Warning

❖ High dosages of enzymes can cause side effects.
❖ If you are allergic to pineapple, you should not take this remedy.
❖ If you have a protein allergy, test your reaction to the preparation by rubbing the tablet on your skin.
❖ Double-check with your therapist as to whether or not you should use this preparation in any of the following cases: blood-thinning disorders, following an operation, pregnancy, or if you take blood-clotting medications.

Recommended dosage: Take one 300 mg capsule of royal jelly once a day over a period of six to twelve months (or one 10 ml liquid ampule of 400 mg royal jelly) or 1,000 mg of flower pollen and 100 mg of propolis once a day over a period of three to six months.

Royal Jelly, Propolis, and Flower Pollen

Bee products are recommended if you are overtaxed physically or mentally, show signs of old age, or have deficiency symptoms. These preparations are extracted from beehives:

Royal jelly is the liquid food of the queen bee and a symbol for vitality, performance power, and life force.

Propolis is the part of the beeswax that contains valuable ingredients, which are effective only if they are released in alcohol.

Flower pollen is carried by the bees back to the hive after they visit male flowers. It contains an abundance of natural ingredients, such as enzymes (see page 91), hormone-like ingredients, antibiotic substances, and substances that raise blood pressure.

Spirulina (Alga Powder)

Spirulina contains as much as 70 percent high-quality protein in addition to many vitamins, minerals, and trace elements. It is an excellent "free radical catcher" (see pages 23–24) and is especially helpful in counteracting constant stress, liver problems, and diabetes. Spirulina also improves mental and physical performance, and prevents you from feeling burnt out.

Parting Words

By reading this book, you have obtained extensive knowledge and thus taken an active step in ridding yourself of your fatigue. Explain what you have learned to your doctor or your natural healing practitioner, and discuss your further therapy with him or her now from a position of greater understanding. In addition, do not hesitate to try the forms of self-treatment recommended here. Having this information about your condition is empowering. And remember, your health is what is most important!

Appendix

Other Possible Diseases

According to the American standard (Center for Disease Control and Prevention), when checking for chronic fatigue syndrome (CFS) the following diseases should be ruled out:

Chronic Problems

• Autoimmune diseases (in which the antibodies or T cells attack the molecules, cells, or tissues of the organism producing them)
• Organ diseases (such as those affecting the heart, liver, or kidneys)
• Tumors (cancer, neoplasia)
• Neurological disturbances (nerve diseases)
• Gland disturbances (endocrine diseases, such as hormonal disturbances of the thyroid, sex glands, suprarenal gland, or pituitary gland)
• Blood diseases (anemia, leukemia, etc.)
• Chronic poisoning (such as poisoning through protective wood varnishes, or quicksilver from amalgams)

Diseases Following Infections

• Chronic hepatitis B or C (liver infections)
• Chronic Lyme disease
• Aids (HIV infection)
• Tuberculosis

Mental Illnesses

• Schizophrenia
• Endogenous depression
• Drug addiction

Additional Possibilities

According to the CFS committee of the German Health Ministry, it is important to rule out the following:

• Malignant tumors
• Autoimmune diseases and other diseases that result from defective granulocytes (a subgroup of the extended blood corpuscles, and also referred to as "cell eaters"), such as connective tissue infections (collagenase), excessive reactions of the immune system in various organs (sarcoidosis), and allergic infections of blood vessels (vasculitis)
• Basic diseases of the blood (hematological diseases), such as anemia, leukemia, and clotting disorders
• Local or systemic (relating to the entire body) infections, hidden abscesses, heart infections (endocarditis, myocarditis), bone-marrow infections (osteomyelitis),
• Borreliosis (caused by ticks) and tuberculosis
• Fungus infections caused by candida, aspergillus, or cryptococcus
• Parasite diseases, such as worms, amebas, or toxoplasma
• AIDS (HIV infection) accompanied by fatigue and severe immune deficiency
• Primary psychiatric diseases, such as psychosis, endogenous depression, or schizophrenia
• Neuromuscular diseases, such as multiple sclerosis (MS), muscular deficiency (myasthenia gravis), muscular diseases caused by infections or metabolic disorders (myopathy)
• Endocrine gland diseases, such as a low level of functioning in the thyroid (hypothyroidism), disturbances of the parathyroid (hypoparathyroidism, mostly after thyroid operations), disturbances of the suprarenal gland (Addison's disease), disturbances of the hormone regulation

centers in the brain (Cushing's syndrome), blood-sugar disease (diabetes mellitus), and metabolic syndromes
• Metabolic changes and electrolyte changes, possibly resulting from vitamin deficiencies (vitamin-D deficiency,

vitamin-B deficiency after stomach operations) or selenium deficiency
• Drug abuse and medication abuse (alcoholism, abuse of painkillers or tranquilizers)

Index

Important Note

Some of the ideas expressed in this book differ from the generally recognized opinions of medical science. It is therefore expected that every reader will use his or her own judgment concerning the extent to which the natural healing remedies that are introduced here can serve as an alternative to conventional medicine.

The following indicators will show you when you have reached the limits of self-treatment and should seek medical assistance:
• If your fatigue lasts for more than three months and does not lessen after a vacation
• If you have any of these symptoms, along with fatigue: weight loss, a pale-looking face, a fever, difficulties breathing while making minor physical efforts (such as walking up stairs), chronic sleep disturbances, severe exhaustion after lunch every day, or chronic diarrhea

About the Author

Vinzenz Mansmann, M.D., is a doctor of both conventional and alternative medicine, a senior consultant of the NaturaMed clinic in Bad Waldsee, Germany, and a specialist in the natural treatment of conditions of fatigue.